Abandoned Child

Also by Toni Maguire

Abandoned Child

Alone and afraid, this is Amy's shocking true
story of survival

TONI
MAGUIRE

with Amy Jones

First published in the UK by John Blake Publishing
An imprint of The Zaffre Publishing Group
A Bonnier Books UK company
4th Floor, Victoria House
Bloomsbury Square,
London, WC1B 4DA
England

Owned by Bonnier Books
Sveavägen 56, Stockholm, Sweden

www.facebook.com/johnblakebooks
twitter.com/jblakebooks

Paperback – 978-1-789-465-93-8
eBook – 978-1-789-465-94-5
Audiobook – 978-1-789-465-95-2

A CIP catalogue of this book is available from the British Library.

Design by www.envydesign.co.uk
Printed and bound in Great Britain by Clays Ltd, Elcograf S.p.A.

1 3 5 7 9 10 8 6 4 2

For each paperback book sold, Bonnier Books UK shall donate 2.5% of its net receipts to the NSPCC (registered charity numbers 216401 and SC037717).

The authors of this work want to show Amy Jones's experience growing up and so you will find language in this book which may be offensive. It is used to show the reality of the author's experience and they and the Publisher would like to add a trigger warning for that here.

This book is a work of non-fiction, based on the life, experiences and recollections of Amy Jones. Certain details in this story, including names and locations, have been changed to protect the identity and privacy of the authors, their family and those mentioned.

John Blake Publishing is an imprint of Bonnier Books UK
www.bonnierbooks.co.uk

Contents

Prologue

I wanted to have my story written down as a book for my daughter to read when she was old enough. There are parts in it that I'm truly ashamed of. Of course, I could leave them out but I won't because my mistakes are a warning, not just to my daughter but to other young people as well. There are people in my story that I should never have made friends with, things I did that I never should have done. Nor should I have stayed with those who tried every trick in an attempt to destroy me.

Towards the end of my story comes the man who I met in my teens. He would describe himself as my ex-partner and, although he is the father of my child, that is not what I would call him – I have other more frightening words in my head about him. If I hadn't learned that he had died, would I have had the courage to put all this in writing? I can't tell you for sure because, after all the years since I left him, his continued presence in my world still terrified me. So, how did I feel when not so long ago I received a letter telling me that he had died of bone cancer when I already knew that he had been ill for some time?

My hands shook as I read that letter. I just about fell backwards on the couch and found myself bursting into tears. But it was not sorrow in any way that caused those tears to dampen my cheeks, it was unbelievable relief.

Finally, I was free.

So, was I his wife?

No, I was his prisoner.

Could I have escaped?

How could a girl who had enjoyed a once-happy childhood become under the control of such a violent and controlling person in the first place? The answer to that question is that there are two types of prison. The ones with bars and locked doors, which make it impossible to walk away. Then there's the other type of prison, where day by day, fear is built and confidence slowly eroded until they become the barrier which prevent the victim from walking through an open door.

So, how does a sociopath like him build that barrier initially? The answer is that they gradually take away every layer of their victim's confidence until there is not a scrap left.

Force her to obey every command until she becomes a human doormat that he can trample on whenever he wishes.

Make her believe that he would find her and beat her almost to death, should she run.

In my story, it's a long journey until I became that victim just at the point when I thought that I was starting to turn my life around. And even longer until, for the sake of my child, I finally managed to leave him.

His outrage and anger when I left him followed me around for over ten years.

Threats came my way.

All those years when I was terrified that he would do as he threatened.

One of these taunts was that he would have my face cut so badly, no man would ever want to look at me again.

Another was that he would take my daughter away from me.

Threats that made me shake each time I received them.

My daughter was not even five when I left him and I did my best to wipe her memories of him away. Even so, she had nightmares about him and those nightmares when she was tiny continued until she was almost in her teens.

It was when she was seventeen and had gone on Facebook that he managed to track us down again. She didn't ever want to see him again. Her memories of him are not that vivid but her dreams were and they came back to haunt her.

So, why did I not go to the police with those taunts and those messages?

Because he made me believe that he and his family had contacts in the force.

Little wonder that him departing this world has changed everything for me. Even so, I have really had to force myself to dig out so many memories and allow them to be printed in this book. It's been a painful process and it's not that easy to have the many wrong steps I took on my journey from child to adult written down for all to read. But I hope it helps someone, anyone. So here goes...

PART ONE

1

Like most other cities, the streets of Leeds are full of people busying themselves shopping during the daytime. Just a few glances at the younger ones gives you an indication of who they are. Strolling around in groups, immersed in deep and earnest conversation, water bottles or takeaway coffees in their hands, tells me they are most probably students. Others, more smartly dressed and walking with purpose and confidence, tell me that they have left university and have now obtained an upmarket job in the thriving businesses in Leeds city centre.

Another glance and I see the *Big Issue* sellers hovering on every corner, asking passers-by to buy one of their magazines. They have been trained to interact with the public and don't feel that they are either jobless or beggars, which gives them some pride, unlike very few of the next group. These are the homeless who sit near the doors to shops, often ignored by passers-by. Over the years I have seen the number of these individuals has increased in the streets of our cities.

There are some who have learnt how to capture the eyes of those walking towards them; they have made sure they have a well-groomed dog with them and that they themselves look neat and presentable. Behind them is their bag containing a few paltry possessions and on their faces a smile with just enough charm to persuade people to drop a few coins into their plastic cups.

Lastly, there are the ones people tend to avoid and act as though they do not even exist, or at least wished they didn't. If they do look at them, their pale faces and skinny frames send the message to everyone nearby them that they are the drug addicts or alcoholics. To many, they represent a threat, appearing dangerous but, to me, they are often just people with a sad past.

Doesn't anyone ever pause to think what happened to make them end up like that? Judging from the way the public hurry past, refusing to look at their thin wrists and grubby outstretched hands or to hear the defeated voices pleading for money for food, I don't think so. It is only the charities that bring food out later in the day. They don't ask questions or ignore those who are dishevelled or dirty, or the addicts. As far as they are concerned, everyone needs to eat to stay alive. Looking at these people on the streets, I can tell that it was not many years ago that they were small children. *Where are their families?* I wonder.

I wish I could get people to think about them differently and not always consider them the scum of the earth. They weren't born that way, were they? I have heard what many people think: that those on drugs are parasites who rob old people of their bags and race away laughing. Even worse, they might follow them home, break in and beat them nearly to death in return for a tenner.

Yes, I must admit, there are those who have committed terrible crimes to feed their addiction. Drugs can sometimes make the person they once were disappear to be replaced by someone who can be frightening and do monstrous things. But let's not blame all of them for that. Many are just helpless and very sick and damaged people from unstable backgrounds. Blame the ones with their pockets stuffed with cash who work so hard at getting them addicted in the first place. Dealers often go for the vulnerable, aware that once they become addicted, they will end up with no family and no support. The addicts who sit shivering in doorways know that the drugs they crave will end up shortening their lives but they no longer care. For them, life is a struggle and all they crave are those brief waves of happiness and oblivion that erase all the dark memories of their troubled pasts.

I myself understand only too well what that feels like. It's when those thoughts enter my head that I see the girl sitting on a bench, her eyes fixed on mine. She has something to tell me, for don't I recognise the ghost of my childhood who refuses to stop haunting?

'Don't let your daughter end up like me,' she murmurs. 'Tell her about my life, how I mixed with the wrong people and lost all of my sense of worth. Show her the marks I made on nearly every part of my body.'

Now that would be a warning to any young person, wouldn't it? I know that children as young at ten are tempted into taking drugs by unscrupulous drug dealers, who they believe are their friends. But they just want to supply drugs so that they can dress in designer gear, wear expensive watches and drive flashy cars. Not all of your teenage daughter's friends are the right ones for her to mix with. It's up to you as a parent to make sure she has the strength to walk away from taking what anyone offers to her. Otherwise it could destroy her and rob her of her future.

The girl smiles and then I find myself looking at an empty bench.

I walk a little further until I come to some steps near a café. Ghost-like, she's there again, sitting on the top step. I know the age of that ghost, it's not quite sixteen. Like many others, she has slipped through the net into homelessness. And I know why that happened: she had no other choice.

The day might be warm to me, but not to her. She's shivering. I see a woman eating a sandwich as she walks past and then, without a glance at the girl, she throws the crusts into the bin at the bottom of the steps. The girl who once was me jumps up, sticks her hand in the bin and pulls them out. It's the only food she is able to eat that day.

When I look again, the woman has disappeared, but the girl is still there.

'You remember that, don't you, or is it another memory you have locked away?' the girl asks.

Of course I remembered that, and the sideways glances that came her way, some pitying but most with distaste and, worst of all, contempt.

'Why, if you saw a girl like that who looked so lost, would

you not help her?' I reflect on her question and ask myself who was there to help me. My mind fills with images of how my early life had been. I was a happy child, living with parents who loved me. Five years later, I was the one sitting on a bench wishing I hadn't fallen out with those who would have made sure that that I was safe and well.

While I was that girl who was homeless, I hoped and prayed that someone would stop and talk to me. Wouldn't they notice that I was barely more than a child and ask what had happened to cause me to sit alone, my bag tucked away behind my feet. I would have told them I had nowhere to go to, that I had to run away. Wouldn't they see the pain in my eyes and offer me help?

But no one came and asked me why I was alone. I had to accept that if I needed help, only I could make it happen.

How much have I told my daughter? Not enough.

Should I?

Yes, I know that I should. She might be shocked, but at least it would have been a warning not to make the same mistakes. How could I let her know everything my early life has taught me? The answer to that is that she can be given the book I want written to read and make of it what she will.

This is the real reason I decided to have my story told.

2

I was ten when my mum passed away. It was Mother's Day 1996; a day I will never forget for it marked the sudden end of all my happiness for the rest of my childhood.

There are so many nights now, when I'm tossing and turning and trying to sleep, that the door in my mind swings open and I'm back there, reliving the day of my mother's funeral. With astonishing clarity, I see the bed my ten-year-old self was curled up in and feel the dampness on her cheeks as she prayed that her mother had not really left her. It was all a nightmare, wasn't it?

Mum's still in hospital, isn't she? Her inner voice refused to accept the reality. *I saw her there only a few days ago. All those nurses and doctors will make her better, won't they? Then she'll come home and everything will go back to how it was before she got ill.*

As my father drew back her bedroom curtains, I can hear his completely expressionless voice telling her that it was time to get up, which meant that it really was true; her mother was never coming home again. She wanted to bury herself deeper in her duvet, to pull it over her head. This was going to be the very worst day of her life. She shuddered as the memory of the night when her aunt sat her down and explained as gently as she could that her mother had died quietly in the hospital bed she had seen her in during her one and only visit.

Aunt Janet was surely heartbroken too for she had just lost the sister she was really close to. How she was able to hide her grief and comfort me, I still don't know. But it was she, not my dad, who wrapped her arms around me and held me close as I sobbed my eyes out. After the tears of grief and anguish made me limp with exhaustion, it was she who managed to help me up the stairs and helped me into my pyjamas and into bed. She fetched me a cup of hot milk and I suspect she might have put something in it to help me sleep because I was strangely drowsy within five minutes. As I lay on my side, she sat beside me, gently stroking my back until I finally drifted off to sleep.

Even now, when I picture that awful day, tears are brimming in my eyes. Out of all of my memories, Mum's funeral is the one thing that never leaves me.

I know that I pretended to be asleep when Dad came into my room that morning. And why was that? To tell the truth, my feelings for him were already changing. Less than a couple of weeks before Mum's death, I would have sat up in bed with a huge grin on my face and my arms out wide, wanting him to give me a kiss and a cuddle – which right up until my mum went into hospital, he always did. But that big jolly man who had shown how much he loved me, the one person I now needed desperately to comfort me, had disappeared the day we left the hospital. In his place was a shadow of himself. The sound of him sobbing like a baby on a daily basis only added to my distress and I was too young to comfort him. Besides, he barely seemed to notice me. Once he had been my hero; the one who rushed into my bedroom when I had a nightmare and told me that no monsters would dare come into my room because he would always fight them off, which always made me giggle. He would brush my hair gently away from my face as he tucked me back into bed, kiss my cheek and wait for a few minutes until I fell back to sleep. But by the day of the funeral, he was no longer the same man.

He managed to do one thing that comforted me during the days between my mum's death and the funeral, which at least kept me busy. Maybe it was to help me or perhaps it was just something he couldn't bring himself to do: he told my aunt and me that instead of having masses of flowers going to the crematorium that within a few days would be dead, we would ask people to donate the money they would have spent on them to Mum's favourite charity, Macmillan Cancer Support. A notice in the local newspaper gave all the details, and friends and family were told much the same thing.

'Your mum would like that, Amy, you know she would,' Aunt Janet and Dad insisted. I must have looked a little disappointed when they said there would be no flowers. But they were right, she would have approved. Mum had been a generous and kind woman who, before she had me, had been a nurse.

'So, Amy, your job is to open up all the letters and cards

that come in, write down how much money is in each envelope and who sent it,' Dad explained before he disappeared
from the house.

I was not expecting the rug under the letter box to be almost
hidden by all those envelopes each and every morning. Once
the kitchen table was cleared, I began to open them, carefully
making a list of the names and noting how many pound notes
were in them or the amounts written on the cheques in the
black book my dad had given me. It was a lot of money. My
next job was to send a thank-you card to each and every
person, which Dad and Aunt Janet would also sign.

I suppose that must have been the first grown-up thing I
had ever done. Up until then I had been quite spoilt by my
parents. I think they both saw me as their little girl, or more to
the point, their beloved only child. Later, I learned that Mum
had two miscarriages before I was born and I was a special,
much-wanted baby. If I wanted something like a new satchel
for school, Dad was only too keen to buy it for me. Maybe
they knew that I would be their only child.

Looking back to the day of the funeral, I realise now that
it was then that everything changed. Without Mum, I was
no longer treated like that precious child. Now there was no
warm voice recounting stories from her childhood or teaching
me how to bake biscuits and cakes while we danced to music
on the radio. No more music and laughter in our home, no
more having a special dress made for me. Without her, the
house became a silent, cold and empty place.

The morning of the funeral, I got myself out of bed, washed
and brushed my teeth, combed my long dark hair and, without

any adult helping me, I somehow managed to tie it into a ponytail. Of course, Aunt Janet would have helped me, but for some reason I wanted to do it all myself. For once she went back to Birmingham, I would have to do it for myself, wouldn't I? Then I pulled on the new black dress that my aunt had bought for me. She had taken my measurements so she could buy it without me there to try it on.

'I don't want to go to the shops,' I had said.

Understanding that I did not want to face it or see any more pity coming in my direction from friends and neighbours, and armed with my measurements, she let me stay behind, opening condolence letters and cards.

Did I have breakfast that morning? I suppose I must have had something, but I can't remember. I do remember Dad was nowhere to be seen. Aunt Janet explained he had gone to the Chapel of Rest to say his last goodbyes before the undertakers prepared to bring Mum to the house. I was so upset I hadn't been asked to go too.

'I wanted to go. I must see her one more time, Aunt Janet. Otherwise, I might not remember her,' I told her.

'No, Amy. I'm not going either. You and I must keep the picture of how she looked the last time you saw her here. I can see her very clearly, with that warm smile of hers and her kind eyes.'

'What would I have seen then, if I had gone with Dad?' I wanted to know.

'She would look peacefully asleep but I know that's not how she would want you to remember her. Your dad and all your aunts and uncles took that decision,' Aunt Janet explained.

I knew there was no point in arguing, but for many years afterwards I regretted not being allowed to say my final goodbyes. When Dad got back, his eyes were red but he said nothing as we all sat at the kitchen table, waiting for the kitchen clock to tick slowly towards the appointed time.

I have a vivid memory of the huge black hearse coming very slowly into our street. Following it was another black car, which was taking all three of us. As we left the house, I saw the coffin with the 'Best Mum' wreath lying on top of it and that was when I lost control. My knees buckled and I felt myself breaking inside. My dad caught my arm and just about carried me to the car behind the hearse, almost pushing me onto the back seat. Janet quickly hopped in beside me and put an arm round me.

'I know this is hard for you, Amy, love,' she said, pushing a wad of tissues into my hand.

The driver opened the other door to the car and Dad came and sat on the other side of me.

'I wanted to go in the car with Mum,' I said. 'I don't understand why I couldn't.'

'It's because the coffin takes up all the rear room, love. And that's why the family always go in separate cars,' Aunt Janet explained.

Groups of neighbours were already outside. As was tradition in our area, they would walk solemnly behind the car all the way to the crematorium, like a black tide following in its wake.

My aunt took my hand then and squeezed it as she said, 'You've been very brave, Amy. Your mum would be so proud of you so just try and think that you want to do the best for her today.'

I nodded, gritted my teeth and bit down on my trembling lip. *I mustn't cry*, I kept telling myself. *I've got to think how Mum would want me to be today.*

As I got out of the car at the crematorium, in my smart new black dress and black beret, the three of us walked towards the chapel. I could hardly believe that so many people were making their way through the gates to say their final goodbyes to Mum – I hadn't realised just how popular she had been and there were a lot of faces I didn't recognise. I knew what everyone must have been thinking and muttering to each other when they looked over at me: 'Poor kid, I feel so sorry for her losing her mum when she's so young.' I could sense their pity in the air all around me.

Dad left us and joined the undertakers and one of my uncles to carry the coffin into the chapel.

'Will we go with Mum too, Aunty Janet?' I asked. I had no experience of funerals and what happened next.

'Yes, we will all enter the chapel once they take your mum inside,' she said.

Once my father came back, we walked inside. I wondered how everyone would fit in, but they all managed, although the place was full from top to bottom. I sat in the front row with all the family, Janet and Dad flanking me. The coffin was on a small stage with black curtains behind it. I can remember feeling completely numb and, apart from listening to all the words of praise for my mother, I hardly took in a word of that service. The worse part for me, which I can still see when

I close my eyes, was the sound of the curtains opening and the coffin with Mum inside it starting to move and slide through into the darkness. As it disappeared from sight, the curtains closed again. The lump in my throat came back and, as we stood, I felt my knees start to buckle again because they were shaking so much.

'Take my arm,' my aunt said gently, no doubt noticing that all the colour must have drained from my face. I was struggling to stand upright and she quickly whispered for me to hold onto her waist. She placed her arm around my shoulder so we could walk out of the chapel together.

Our family group stood together outside and thanked everyone for coming. All I wanted was to get away from them. I could feel the tears trying to force their way out. *No, I mustn't cry, not now anyway*, I kept telling myself.

It was when I saw my headteacher, Mr Vasey, walking towards me that I nearly broke down again. I felt his arms go around me as he gave me a hug.

'I just want my mummy back,' I kept telling him, my body wracked with sobs.

In my heart of hearts, I knew that as soon as my mother's body had disappeared behind the curtain, with it had gone my childhood.

3

So what was my life like after the funeral? Empty. It was as though grief had small sharp teeth that gnawed at my mind until the pain became so intense, I could hardly move. When I closed my eyes, pictures of the very last time I had seen Mum tormented me as each one pushed itself inside my head. It was the happy times and not those last memories that I wanted to dwell on. I wish I could have put a barrier in my mind to stop the pictures of Mum's last day being foremost in my memories, for they were too distressing for a ten-year-old to deal with. To say I missed her nearly every moment of the day would be an understatement, though even now I can't find the right words to describe how I felt then. Worse than numb is all I can remember. I didn't want to go out, I didn't want to talk to anyone and, most of all, I didn't want to have people trying to be kind or to comfort me.

Our neighbours did their best to help us in our grief. They took it in turns to bring round cooked meals. However appetising they appeared, neither Dad nor I were hungry. To us, food was just something we had to put in our mouths because we knew our bodies needed it. We pushed it around on our plates and ate in silence, for what could we say?

After Mum died, I felt as if I was living in an empty house with none of the atmosphere that had been there before remaining. It became even bleaker for me when my aunt left. I understood she had to go back to her family, but she was someone else I was going to miss. I wanted to cling to her and tucked my head under her chin like a small child would do as she hugged me goodbye. But I didn't do that, even though I craved the support and affection that my parents had always given me. I no longer saw myself as a little girl. Aunt Janet told me that she would ring, we could chat, and then she promised she would be back soon to see how we were doing. If she had told me a date when that would be, I would have counted off the days.

I can remember now just how forlorn I felt standing at the doorway as I watched her climb into her car and drive off. The last embers of warmth in our house had left with her. She and Mum were always chatting on the phone together, sometimes their calls would last for hours. When I heard the hoots of laughter, it would make me smile. Tears slid down my face as the car disappeared from sight. Without her, there was no one to comfort me, despite Dad standing there right by my side, politely waving goodbye. As the car turned the corner he closed the door, went into the sitting room, sat down on his usual chair and opened the newspaper. I didn't know if he was reading it or just hiding behind the pages. Anything seemed preferable to him than having to talk to me.

Ever since that final visit to the hospital, he had done his best to ignore me, or so it seemed. Our closeness was gone – in fact, I'm convinced that it was slowly seeping away since the day the ambulance was called.

Mum's best friend, Anne called round to see us. She told Dad that, if he was going back to work, I could come to hers after school and stay there until he came home.

'It would not be good for Amy to return each day to an empty house,' she explained.

Dad just murmured, 'OK,' and perhaps as an afterthought added a muffled, 'Thanks.'

I was certainly grateful for that offer but, even though I had known Anne's children all of my life, I still found it impossible to join in and play with them after Mum died. I used the excuse of homework to sit and stare at the blurred pages of a book. Thankfully, Anne never noticed that I did not turn the pages.

Once the arrangement started, I didn't mention to Anne how Dad was being towards me. There didn't seem much point and I was still suffering with my own grief. But after a couple of weeks, Dad did surprise me by saying he was going to the working men's club on the Saturday – a club that, although it had that name, was often full of families at the weekend.

'Thought it would be a change to go out and I think it would do you good too if you come as well, Amy.'

'Yes, thanks, Dad,' I managed to say because it was not somewhere that, without Mum, I really wanted to go to.

I did my best to make myself look smart that evening, not

that he made any comment when I came down the stairs and saw him freshly showered and shaved, wearing his tweed jacket and grey trousers. I suppose, when we walked into the place, people immediately thought that he was doing his best to look after me and being there might succeed in cheering me up a little. They got that wrong. I hated being there; to me it was too full of memories. Only a few weeks earlier, I had been sitting in between Mum and Dad with people coming over to chat to us and Mum telling jokes, which made us all laugh. Now there was no laughter or even much conversation as I sat with Dad sipping a Coca-Cola while he knocked back pints of beer. Instead of feeling it was a cheerful place, I could sense thick waves of pity coming in our direction. Of course, a lot of people did come over to our table, the first one being Mum's best friend, Anne, and they all tried to be as nice and friendly to us as they could. Not that Dad responded much, though I suppose he must have tried a little.

I wonder if anyone noticed that there was no warmth coming from him towards me. No arm round my shoulder, nor was I leaning against him. I suppose they just saw a grief-stricken man trying his best to give his daughter a pleasant evening. But then they would not have known why his affection for me had disappeared the night before Mum died and what happened when he had taken me to the hospital. That, as well as the funeral, is another recollection which over the years has remained in memory, sharp and acutely clear.

That evening, I suspect Mum must have asked to see me. I guess she knew as well as he did that she was dying and that it was his duty to let me see her for the last time.

Only then was I told the truth about why she was in hospital and not at home, ill in bed. It was when Anne turned up at school and explained to me why she had come to take me to her house. When I saw her walking towards me when school finished, I was pleased to see her. She put her arm round my shoulders as she said, 'Nothing to worry about, Amy, it's just that I've come to bring you over to my house. Your Mum's got flu and neither your mum nor dad want you to catch it so we think it's better if you stay with us for a few days. I've been over to your house and picked up a few of your clothes from your bedroom. Hope you don't mind.'

'No, I don't mind at all,' I told her, because I loved staying with her. Her house was almost like a second home to me. Which is why I didn't think that her coming to fetch me was unusual. After all, when I was a little younger and my parents were going out for dinner together, instead of having a babysitter, I would go to hers and stay the night. As she and my mum had been friends for years, her children and I had played together since we were little more than toddlers. That day I was happy to be going with her. I think the only question I asked was, 'How long before Mum gets better?' But then why would I not have believed what she had told me? I didn't even think to ask any questions, why would I at that age?

When I think back now it all makes sense that, when I stayed in Anne's home, there were a few odd thing happening that at the time I didn't give much thought to. Such as when there was a knock at the door and Anne rushed to open it and I could hear adult's voices whispering on the doorstep. Not that I took much notice because I was probably looking at comic books or trying to do my homework. Had I been a little older, I might have wondered why they were whispering. I realise now that they had to be saying something they didn't want me to hear.

I did notice, though, that when I walked into the sitting room when Anne had visitors, they all stopped talking, but then I knew that adults sometimes do that. Like when they talk about problems with their children or their husbands and don't want us to hear about it. It took less than a week before I would understand what it was that they had been talking about and what it was they had wanted to hide from me.

Those two days with Anne were the last ones of me being a giggling, happy little girl. The next day, Dad arrived at the school early in the afternoon. He must have told the headmaster his reason for collecting me when he sought his permission to take me home. All I thought at the time was that it was great to be getting out of school before the end of the day, he and Mum must have planned a treat for me. Especially when he told me that my mother's sister, Aunt Janet, had driven all the way up from Birmingham to stay with us. Was that because it was Mother's Day on Sunday, I asked?

I think Dad managed to wait until we were back in the house before he told me why I had been picked up from school. If only I hadn't asked what we were doing on Mother's Day, maybe he wouldn't have stopped the car abruptly and blurted everything out, which reduced me to tears.

'Look, Amy, we had decided not to tell you straight away, but your mum's not at home with flu, she's in hospital. She's had a brain haemorrhage and she's asking to see you. That's why I came to the school to pick you up. We have to go and see her today.'

My voice was already trembling when I asked tentatively, 'What's a brain haemorrhage?'

'It means there's something inside her head that has made it bleed,' he told me. 'But it's a really good hospital and I know she's going to get better. And then we'll have her back home.'

A hard knot formed in my stomach: it was fear swirling into my mind. I began to cry for there was nothing in the tone of his voice or in his body language that was reassuring. Without saying anything more, he turned on the engine and drove us back to the house. It might only have taken five minutes but, to me, it felt it as if it was ages before we reached the road running through our small village and I could see the familiar golden cornfields sweeping down towards the houses.

Mum had told me that they had chosen to live there because the village, being nice and peaceful, was an ideal place to bring up children. I sat in the car and thought about the last weekend when the bluebells in the wood behind our house had bloomed and Mum and I walked there to admire their beauty. That made me all the more tearful, but it was when I glanced at Dad and saw tears trickling down his cheeks that I couldn't believe I was seeing right. I had always regarded him as a big, tough man. Like so many of his friends and acquaintances, he had worked in the mines for over 20 years. If I had been frightened before by what he had told me, I was now petrified. I had never seen him like this and the fact that he was tearful told me that, whatever was wrong with Mum, I had every reason to be concerned.

It was that thought that made me realise that the reason Mum's sister Janet had left her family on the Mother's Day weekend and driven from Birmingham without notice meant that Mum must be very ill indeed. Almost as soon as Dad parked the car in front of our house, the one where I was born, I saw some of the neighbours walking towards us. I should think he regretted being in a small village where everyone knew everyone's business. All we wanted was to get in the house as quickly as possible.

'You OK, John?' one of the men asked as Dad got out of the car.

Even I could tell that he wasn't OK.

Without even looking at him, Dad just muttered, 'Yes.'

'How's Mary doing?' another wanted to know. To which he replied, 'All right,' before bounding up the path, leaving me behind unbuckling my seat belt to scramble out. I saw the pity in their eyes. Whatever had happened to Mum was really serious and they knew. They would have seen the ambulance arrive and heard the siren as it took off as fast as it could, with her inside. Maybe that's the reason why, even as a teenager, I never liked that pitying look when it was turned towards me. Today, I still don't cope well with people feeling sorry for me.

Like Dad, I, too, rushed away from those neighbours. They might have been kindly but I couldn't cope with their pity. Janet opened the door Dad had slammed behind him, put an arm around me and drew me up against her to give me a hug.

'Come into the kitchen, love, and I'll get us something to eat,' she told me.

Strangely enough, as soon as I walked into the hall with

everything going through my head, I noticed immediately how immaculate our house was. Certainly, it would not have been Dad who had made it so tidy – Janet must have been pretty busy since she got there. A pot of tea was quickly made, which she poured into mugs, and then stirred some sugar into one of them before placing it in front of me.

'Look, Amy,' she said as soon as she sat down, 'I know how upsetting this is for all of us but I doubt your mum ever told you that six years ago I had exactly the same problem as her and I was also rushed into hospital. When she got the call telling her where I was, she rushed down to me the same day and she was by my side as I fought for my life.'

'No, she never said. So where was I?' I wanted to know.

'You were only four. I had a friend babysit you in my house while your mum was visiting me. My husband arranged that. Anyway, what I'm trying to tell you is that I'm still here!' she told me.

'When am I going to see Mum?'

'Your dad is taking you soon.'

'Aren't you coming too?'

'No, sweetheart, I've been already and they don't like too many visitors in the special ward she's in. What I need to ex-plain, easier than your dad probably can, is that your mum will look a bit different than you are used to. She also has all different machines that's she's attached to, which are helping her. The doctors and nurses are doing everything they can. I know it's not going to be easy for you to see her like that, but she wants you to go. So, you'll have to be brave for her sake. Can you manage to look cheerful when you see her?'

'I won't cry, if that's what you mean.'

'No, I didn't think you would. You don't just look like your mum when she was young, you have her strength too. I can tell because I can remember what she was like when she was your age.'

'Now, let me get you both a toasted sandwich,' she added quickly as Dad walked into the kitchen.

He hardly said a word as he sat down to eat, just swallowed what he could manage and, the moment I had finished my toastie, he stood up.

'Time to go, Amy,' he announced as he walked into the hall.

'Now remember what I said, love, don't let your mum seeing you looking upset,' Janet told me.

'I won't,' I promised as she gave another quick hug.

Although I had made that promise and I was determined not to show anything but a cheerful face, it didn't stop me feeling sick with nerves. Aunt Janet had also told me that Mum might be asleep when we got to the hospital, but it was that word 'machines' that really got to me. *Just what were they doing to her?* I wanted to ask Dad why she needed those machines and, had it been a few days earlier, I might have done so, but instinct told me it was best not to ask. He had hardly spoken to me since I came home. As he drove out of the village and along the roads leading to the hospital, he was concentrating on the road ahead.

I felt even more nervous when we drew up to what seemed like a huge hospital, parked the car and walked silently through the hospital doors. For once, Dad took my hand – I think it must have been to give us both strength. The lift took us to Mum's ward and we went straight in. A nurse told us that she was sleeping but not deeply, so if we sat there for a while she would probably wake up. What I noticed straight away was the silence: no chatter coming from the patients, the curtains were drawn around some of the beds, and through them I could see the shadowy silhouettes of visitors sitting quietly.

As Dad had been there before, he led me straight to Mum's bed and the nurse drew back the curtain. Seeing her lying so still made that lump enter the back of my throat again and my eyes pricked with tears, which I was determined not to let fall. She looked so tiny lying there. Just a few days ago I had been chatting and laughing while she, the robust woman I loved so much, cooked supper for the three of us. I realised that was the evening before Anne came to the school to tell me Mum had flu. How could she have changed in just three days? She was almost as pale as the bed sheets tucked around her. I could see she was asleep for her eyes were closed and, with those thick dark lashes of hers, her face looked even more pallid. Was I supposed to just sit there in the hope that she would wake? When I glanced around me, I saw more pitying looks, this time coming from the nurses. It made me decide that I hadn't come to the hospital to sit still and say nothing to my mother.

I did my best to swallow away that lump in my throat, for hadn't I promised Aunt Janet not to let her see how upset I was, a promise that I was doing my best to keep? Before anyone could tell me to wait until she woke, I opened my mouth and said as gently as possible, 'Hello, Mummy.'

I heard Dad give an indignant gasp but before he could

tell me off, we could see that she had recognised my voice and that had made her eyes flicker and open. For just a few seconds a smile came onto her face as she looked at me. Then everything changed. Her smile disappeared and I saw fear in her eyes as she glanced over my shoulder towards Dad.

'Amy, who's that man with you?' Her voice had a note of anger in it, which filled me with such surprise that I could not answer immediately. It was then that she began to shout, which got the nurses running to her bedside. 'Get away from my daughter! Get away from me too!' she yelled with her remaining strength. She meant Dad; her husband of 17 years and she hadn't recognised him. At least she recognised me. I heard her voice change to a confused whisper as she said to the nurse who was bending over her, 'Where am I?' and the nurse replied softly that she was being cared for in hospital. It was then that Mum choked out sobbingly the saddest words I had ever heard from her: 'I want to go home now, my daughter has come to get me.'

I didn't know what to do and I looked at Dad helplessly, hoping he would say something reassuring. Instead, he gave me such a black glare that I almost stumbled backwards. To me, it was a look of pure hatred and it was coming in my direction. It was something I have never forgotten and it was the last straw of the day. The tears I had tried to block since I had first seen Mum were now running down my face.

'All right, Amy, time for us to go. Seeing you has obviously upset your mum.'

With that, he took hold of my arm firmly, told the nurse he would come back later and marched me briskly out.

The drive back home from the hospital was not only filled with silence but, as an adult, I now know that what was in the air was hate. Every time I spoke, I was ignored or told I'd done enough harm for the day. I couldn't understand it, was it not a good sign that Mum remembered me?

He clearly did not think so.

4

How long does it take that huge ball of grief to bring us down completely? In my case it took six months. And when did my life begin to change? It had started immediately. Right from the beginning, there were those who had the power to change the girl I was into a very different one. Not that anyone, including myself, realised it for some time.

During those six months, I don't think there was anyone who considered that my grief in losing Mum still hadn't hit me completely. From what I remember, it seemed that everyone, including Mum's friends, believed that I was coping with her death a little more each day and for a while I must have believed that hypothesis too. I know during that time I often felt I needed to be alone so that I could go back in time and dwell on those special memories of Mum and I together. I would lie on my bed, close my eyes and then run those visual images, picture by picture, through my mind. My breath would slow and somewhere from deep inside me would come the pictures.

The one that always came first was the last time we were all out together as a family. It was only two weeks before she died. Dad had taken us to Cleethorpes for the day. It was a place that we all loved going to, even if the sea was grey and cold and the donkeys weren't there offering small children rides because trade would be too slow. There were plenty of other things we enjoyed doing, although to our delight, by mid-morning the grey clouds slid away, leaving a pale blue sky behind. The sun came out and shone its golden rays on the pale sand that stretched for miles. A good place to walk along for a while, as it was deserted except for a few dog walkers.

I noticed that Mum seemed more enthusiastic about being there than usual. I didn't think about it much then, but she seemed to be making herself enjoy the day more than she normally did. Now I wonder, considering what seemed like high spirits plus all the affection she showed me that day, if she had a premonition that something was going to happen; something that would separate her from us forever. Or was she remembering her sister's time in hospital, hovering between life and death, and wondered if that was something that might run in the family? Whatever it was, I will never know the answer. I can still hear her voice in my head saying, 'What a beautiful young girl you are, Amy,' and I could see the love she felt for me in her eyes as she stroked my hair and pushed some windblown tendrils behind my ears then gave me such a bear hug that it made me nestle up to her.

After our walk on the beach, with Mum assuring us that all that fresh air was good for us, we strode over to the arcade where she and Dad enjoyed playing the machines. Whoops filled the air when one of them won. 'Here, my chicken licken,' Mum said to me with a wide smile as she handed over a bag full of 2p coins. I spent nearly all of them in the drop machines, where I pressed away at the button that made the claw move. There was a small black and white stuffed dog that I wanted, which I finally got. I still have it, as a token of the day, though it's pretty shabby now.

'Time for lunch, Amy. How about fish and chips?' Dad asked.

As we had them every time we visited, I giggled as I answered, 'Yes, Dad.'

After all, we had all agreed that Cleethorpes' chips were the best ones in the area.

We were sitting down on the café's wooden chairs when Mum began to talk about our summer holiday. That year it was Turkey.

'The food there is wonderful,' she told me, 'and there's a huge swimming pool in the hotel. There's one for the small children, but you're such a good swimmer, you won't need that, will you, Amy?'

'I shouldn't think so,' I replied with confidence. 'I can do two lengths now, Mum.'

Mum had already shown me pictures of the part of Turkey we were going to. I thought it looked beautiful, and as for the hotel, the brochure showed a luxurious place, but then, with the benefit of two salaries, Mum and Dad always chose such good holidays. Like her, I was really looking forward to going abroad and being assured of hot and sunny weather.

That conversation made me even more enthusiastic and I

began to count the days, not just to my summer break from school, but to the morning we would all get on the plane that would take us all the way to Turkey.

Mum talking about the holiday again made me feel relieved, because the pair of them were smiling at each other and recently I had been worried. They didn't know that I had heard their rows; they might have thought that I was sound asleep when Dad staggered into the house late, which I was. But not deeply enough not to be woken up by loud and angry shouting in the hallway when Mum confronted him. It was then that I did what many children do – I crept silently out of my room and listened to them with my sharp little ears straining to take in their words.

I soon learned that it was not only about his drinking and how he came home stinking of booze, but also that she couldn't stand how he acted when he was drunk. All that shouting and swearing was muffled but her words, 'I'm not going to put up with it any longer,' were loud and clear.

'That's not the way I want my daughter brought up. I don't want her to have a drunk for a father. It's not good for any child to lose all respect for their parents. Anyway, you look a mess – take a look at yourself in the mirror.'

That was enough to make me crawl back into my room. I knew better than to get caught.

Then there was another time when what I heard made me shake. Dad had arrived home drunk again. I could hear his voice slurring as he tried to make his excuses. And then I heard Mum's voice, cold as ice as she said, 'Don't think I won't leave you, John. I need to think of my daughter as well as myself.'

Now I believe that he planned the holiday and the day out in Cleethorpes as part of an attempt to make things up with Mum. I have no doubt that he loved her, as he did me, but it was a love that did not take long to crumble.

Those are just some of my memories but there are so many more that I also cling to.

5

But now I want to get to the part of my story where Dad and I did go on that holiday, even though Mum had died. I thought there was no way he'd want to go so soon after her death. Surely most husbands would cancel the family holiday? You'd think so, right? But he was adamant that Mum would have wanted us both to go, and besides, it was too late to get a refund and they had saved up for the trip.

It was the start of the school holidays and he kept saying, 'We're a team now, Amy, just you and me.' Which was not exactly how I saw us. But still, I did my best. My birthday was on 24 June 1985. He asked if I wanted a party, but I said no – I couldn't have coped without Mum being there. Instead, he took me out for a meal and then told me what my present was: a brand-new wardrobe of holiday clothes, which I would get on the Saturday.

'Anne told me you had grown a lot since last holidays and offered to have a look at some of the hems to see if she could let them down. I told her not to bother, said you could have all new things instead. I mean everything, Amy – swimsuits, shorts, T-shirts and a couple of nice dresses. You'd better have some new sandals as well. How does that sound?'

I could hardly speak, I was so surprised. Dad had never mentioned my clothes before, but then that was Mum's job. I must have managed to say something that made me sound grateful. After all, what eleven-year-old wouldn't be excited about a whole new suitcase of holiday clothes?

Anne arrived early on the Saturday morning and announced, 'Amy, I hope you have a list of what you want for your holiday in Turkey. I've made one anyhow and your dad told me what he thought you would need.'

Dad handed her a thick envelope of cash, saying, 'If you have time, Anne, why don't you treat yourselves to lunch or a nice tea using this?' And with a flourish, out came another envelope of cash.

'Well, thanks, John, that would be nice,' she said.

Later, she mentioned quite a famous old-fashioned place that did wonderful cakes. My appetite still wasn't good, but the word 'cake' almost made my mouth water.

'Let's begin with swimming costumes, shorts and T-shirts,' said Anne as we made our way out of the house and got into her car to drive to the shopping centre. 'That's the daytime stuff and then you'd better have a couple of dresses for when your dad takes you out in the evenings.'

By the time we had chosen all those clothes and were laden down with bags, our last stop was to buy me some sandals and a new pair of trainers. 'Might need them if you're doing a lot of walking,' Anne told me. 'And we've forgotten a cardigan and some new underwear and pyjamas.'

It was when we finally left the last shop that, for one fleeting moment, I thought I saw Mum across the road. She was dressed in one of her nicest coats and walking a short distance in front of us. Without thinking, I shouted out, 'Mum!' Seeing I was just about ready to run after the woman, Anne caught hold of my arm. I couldn't stop myself bursting into tears and, feeling the tension in my body, Anne put her arms around me.

'Amy, try and take a deep breath now.' She led me to a seat and sat with her arm about me. In between gulping sobs, I tried to slow my breathing until I felt a little calmer.

I heard her saying softly, 'I recognised that coat too, Amy. You know, don't you, that it was just seeing it that made you think that the woman wearing it was your mum?'

'She loved that coat,' I sighed. 'She bought it last year when we were in Italy.'

Of course, I knew what had happened to all her clothes: Dad had taken them all to the charity shops. And that woman, seeing a bargain, had probably snapped the coat up. Anne didn't say what I believe she must have been thinking, why on earth hadn't he taken them to another town? Surely, he didn't want his daughter seeing them in the charity shop windows? But then he was not a man who thought too deeply about how not to upset anyone. At least that was what she told me a long time later and, by that time, I already knew it was true.

You might wonder why I've written a whole chapter about a holiday. One where, unexpectedly, I did manage to enjoy myself. I'll give you the reason now: it shows the child I was then, not the one that so much of my story is about. Looking back, I can see that, if what took place after the holiday hadn't happened, I might have grown up to become a very different person.

6

Once the day of the start of our holiday came and all our clothes and whatever else we needed was packed in the suit-cases that Dad took into the hall, I felt such a wave of sadness. It was only a year ago when the three of us had been in the same place for the same reason, while we waited for the taxi to take us to the airport. Mum had bustled around checking that everything was packed and that she had the tickets, pass-ports, currency and credit cards in her handbag. After all that was done and we closed the front door behind us, how happy she looked. When Dad had brought all the cases down and placed them by the door, she put her arms around me and gave me a tight squeeze.

'We're going to have a fun time over there, aren't we? But then we always have great holidays together, don't we?' she said.

'Yes,' I replied, for that was true: we did.

Every year my parents would choose a different country for us to visit. The three of us would sit together and look at brochures, discussing the pictures of hotels and their swimming pools until we made up our minds on which package to book, though frankly I would have been happy with any one of them. While we stood in our hall that day, Mum and I were really excited at the thought that, within a short time, we would be stepping into a plane which would land in another country.

But this year, the change in the atmosphere when it was only the two of us waiting to leave was huge. I know Dad was doing his best to appear cheerful, but he couldn't convince me that he wasn't missing Mum as much as I was. In a way, I wished we weren't going – I could hardly believe that we could have anything like the fun we had when Mum was there. Whatever I muttered to Dad about looking forward to going with him, it simply wasn't true.

7

I couldn't help it, I just didn't want to go. Not one thing leading up to the holiday made me happy. Even that day with Anne when we went shopping for holiday clothes didn't cheer me up. This time it was only me who needed new things whereas a year earlier, Mum and I had gone shopping together. Despite quite a full wardrobe, she, too, was keen to buy the occasional new dress and would always pop her head around the changing room door to ask my opinion. In between shopping, she would take me to a café, where we sat and chatted about the place we were going to.

As I've said, each year it would be a different country – 'Good for your geography,' Mum would say, laughing, as she chattered about all the sights we were going to see. She enjoyed doing her research and made a list of places of interest in the area we were going to and what their local food delicacies were. She loved tasting new foods and, when we returned home, she would try to cook those dishes we had liked best.

I knew when I set off with Anne that she understood how much I must have been missing Mum. She did everything she could to make me feel better about going away and kept telling me that the Turkish beaches where we were going were just about the best ones. 'The Turkish food is wonderful too,' she said.

I managed to smile and say, 'That's great,' but what I didn't tell her was that, without Mum, whatever food I ate – and I ate a lot for comfort by that time – tasted like sawdust. Fond as I was of Anne, nothing we did that day was the same as being with Mum – if anything, it made me miss her even more.

While Dad and I waited in the hall for our taxi, I could feel her absence every second until it came. When we heard the taxi draw up, we glanced at each other. All he said was, 'It's here, let's go,' and he opened the front door, grabbed hold of our cases, placed them on the step and locked the door. 'You can carry your little bag,' he told me as he picked up the others and put them in the taxi.

It was when the car began to move that I pondered Dad's silence. I decided that he must have the same feelings about Mum not being there as I had. He hardly spoke at all on that journey and I had nothing to say either. Once we arrived at the airport and Dad peeled off enough notes, including a tip for the driver, he placed our luggage on the trolley. With me following him, he walked quickly to the check-in. Dad showed them our passports and tickets, which he had stashed in a special wallet. Our luggage was underweight, so no problem there and it didn't take us long to go through to the departure lounge.

'That was pretty easy, wasn't it?' Those were just about

the first few words to come out of his mouth since we left the house. 'Would you like a drink and a biscuit, Amy? You didn't have any breakfast.'

'Yes, please,' I said – I needed something to nibble on because, tasteless or not, swallowing food calmed me down.

'You stay with our hand luggage and keep our seats,' he told me and then walked over to the coffee shop.

He came back with a milky drink for me and a KitKat. I could see his drink was a lot stronger.

Boarding the plane and finding our seats was easy. Not long after take-off, trolleys with food and drink started coming down the aisles. For once I found myself tucking into what was on my cardboard plate. Not long after that I must have dozed off. I remember hearing Dad's voice saying, 'Hey, Amy, wake up! We're landing in a few minutes. Have a look out of the window and see how sunny it is.'

I pressed my head against the window and there was the sea sparkling under the sun's golden rays. All around us I could hear the other passengers' excitement at finally being there, and wasn't the sea beautiful? I could see it was and the blueness of it made me feel a little more cheerful.

Once we had collected our luggage and went through customs, Dad spotted a man holding a large sign with the name of our hotel on it.

'He must be our driver,' Dad said almost cheerfully. 'And he's certainly bang on time. Let's go up to him.'

As we walked over, I noticed that a few other people were heading in the same direction. The driver was all smiles and spoke reasonably good English. When our group had all arrived, he made sure he hadn't left anyone behind, counted heads and checked paperwork to ensure that we were all booked into the hotel. He told us to follow him out to where the minibus was parked. Along with the others staying at our hotel, we wheeled our trolleys out to where our driver was parked. Within a few minutes all of us were seated comfortably inside. A few couples introduced themselves, not that I can remember all their names now. I can recall the ones who sat on seats near us – Dawn and Craig – who told us their names and then chatted away for most of the short journey.

I heard Dad say, 'Why don't we meet up for a drink in the bar before we have dinner?'

'Good idea, John,' said Craig. 'I was just about to suggest that but you got in first. Let's say thirty minutes before dinner, does that suit you, and you too, Amy?'

At this, I couldn't help but smile.

'Yes,' I answered, as did Dad.

The driver had been using a microphone to point out areas of interest to us as he drove and, in no time at all, the minibus slowed and I heard the driver's voice announcing that we had arrived. I just about gasped with pleasure when I clambered out and saw the hotel, our home for a whole two weeks. With its brightly coloured balconies and beautiful grounds with a mass of stunning plants, I was just about awestruck: to me, it was the loveliest place I had ever seen. From the remarks Craig and Dawn were making about it being even more beautiful than in the brochure, I seemed to be not the only one who was impressed.

How I wished Mum was there. How she would have loved

it. I couldn't help but think that she, too, would have been just as overwhelmed as I was if she had been standing beside me.

'Not only is this the hotel very attractive, but it's also very well situated,' Dad told me. 'There won't be any traffic noise coming through our bedroom windows and keeping us awake and it's just a ten-minute walk to the sea. You'll like walking on the beach tomorrow morning, won't you, love?'

'Yes, Dad,' I said, making myself smile up at him. It really was lovely there, I told myself, and he clearly wanted me to enjoy this holiday, even though it must have been difficult for him as well.

Once inside, I had a peek through the large French windows and saw the enormous pool that all the hotel residents could use. That really pleased me because swimming was one thing I had loved since I was very young. It was Dad who had taught me on our first holiday as a family. He always said I had taken to it like a duck to water. It was on another holiday that I had also learnt to dive. Dad thought of a game where he threw coins into the pool, which I could keep if I collected them underwater – I don't think I missed one.

Anyway, the moment that I saw the pool with its tall diving board, I decided that I was going to leap from it.

The staff at the hotel couldn't have been friendlier either. After we had checked in, a porter came over, placed all our luggage on a trolley and pushed it into the lift before accompanying us to our rooms. As they were next door to each other, Dad said I could have a look at both and choose whichever one I wanted. I simply loved the first one I saw. With its really comfortable-looking bed, which had plenty of pillows on it, a wardrobe filled with loads of hangers and a built-in dressing table with a hairdryer, it couldn't be better, I thought, as I walked over to the window to admire the balcony where I could stand out and admire the pool and the grounds.

'I'll have this one, Dad, it's amazing!' I said gratefully.

'Good, pleased you like it. You can sort out your luggage, have a shower and change for dinner. I'll knock on the door in about forty-five minutes,' he told me after glancing at his watch. 'Then we can have a walk round the grounds before meeting up with Craig and Dawn in the bar.'

I felt quite grown-up when, for the first time on a holiday, I unpacked, hung up my clothes and chose which dress to wear for dinner. At least with them all being new, none of them brought back memories. I think Anne had advised Dad to let me get all new ones because Mum used to make quite a few of my things. And without saying anything to me, with my newly acquired nibbling habit, she had noted that I had not just grown a little taller, but was looking a little tubby.

I chose a pretty blue and white striped dress and laid it out on the bed before I had my shower. The hotel's flowery scented body wash and shampoo made me feel fresh and clean as well as wide awake after my journey.

I got ready and within a few minutes I heard Dad tapping at my door before he walked in, wearing a T-shirt and a light-coloured pair of trousers.

'You're looking very nice,' he said. 'Now let's have a look round the grounds.'

Down we went and stepped out through the open French doors, where the pool was located. A few people were still stretched out on the loungers and a couple who had arrived with us were already swimming in the clear blue water.

'Can't wait to get in there too,' I told Dad, who laughed and said, 'Me too, Amy. This place has such a peaceful feel to it.'

When we moved away from the pool to explore the gardens, there was the mesmerising scent of the flowers. All that beauty around me began to lift my depression. As we walked back, I could see the balcony outside my room. It made me feel happy that I had one all to myself, for I had always shared a room with Mum and Dad on previous holidays. Looking back, I was young to have a room of my own – I wouldn't be in different rooms without my kids, or certainly not without an adjoining door, but I didn't think anything of it then. In fact, I was grateful to have my own space.

'Come on, we'll go to the bar now. It's time to meet up with Dawn and Craig,' said Dad.

As I walked beside him through the hotel to the the restaurant, I thought that was really pretty as well. There were flowers everywhere and the whole place was light and airy.

'Hi there, you two,' said Craig as he and Dawn walked in just as Dad was ordering drinks for us – 'Lemonade, Amy?'

'I can make your daughter a non-alcoholic cocktail,' the barman offered.

'All right, I think you'll like that, Amy. And what can I get you two?' said Dad.

'Cocktails, but we'll have a little more alcohol in ours,' they said in unison.

Having Dawn and Craig with us in the bar helped a lot.

I think Dad must have managed to quickly tell them when I was getting ready why it was just the two of us on holiday. That would explain why, apart from being really friendly to me, they never asked any questions about my home life or even what I liked most at school. They did tell us they had not been married long and that they wanted to have a couple more holidays before they started a family, which seemed to amuse Dad – 'Yes, babies shrieking on the plane is never that great. Not that Amy ever did that, thank goodness.'

After that, the subject was changed and the pair talked about places they wanted to see in Turkey. There was one that they described, a big spice and shopping bazaar, that made me want to go too. Dad also looked interested, so I knew we would be going. After another round of cocktails that Craig ordered, we all went into the dining room to have dinner together and that was the start of us doing a lot of things together.

Somehow it seemed easier for Dad and me to have other people who had never known Mum around us. There was laughter at that table, something I hadn't heard much of since her death. Arrangements were made for us to go sightseeing together and, to my delight, a trip to the bazaar was arranged for the following day.

'Lots of lovely things to see and buy there from what I've heard,' said Dawn. 'I'm definitely planning to go shopping. Now, Amy, how about us girls having a morning at the pool? I gather you're a real water baby. We can go to the bazaar later in the day when it's a bit cooler and we've had enough sun. Would you like that?'

A wide smile stretched my cheeks as I said, 'I would, I really would. How did you know I love swimming?'

'Your dad told me. He said you were really good at it.'

'Yes, I do love swimming and that pool is the best one I've ever seen in a hotel.'

'And how about we find a good Turkish restaurant to go to that night? The food here is good but Dawn and I always like to try little local places too,' said Craig, smiling.

'Good idea, I'm up for that,' agreed Dad. 'OK, Amy?'

I couldn't help it, but I was beginning to feel sleepy. Noticing that I was having difficulty keeping my eyes open, Dad said, 'I think it's bedtime for you, Amy.' He stood up and, holding his hand out for me to take, walked me to the lift and up to my room. It struck me then that his mood was so much better than it had been since that scene in the hospital and he even gave me a hug and told me to sleep well.

I crawled into bed and I must have fallen asleep straight away, for the next thing I remember was the sun's rays coming through the curtains to rest warmly on my face. My eyes flickered open and for a moment I wondered where I was. *In Turkey, you idiot*, my inner self told me. *And that's sun telling you to get up and get down to the pool*. That was enough to make me push my legs out of the bed and get up. On went my swimsuit and over the top went a pair of shorts and a tee. Finally, I slipped my feet into a pair of sandals.

Better let Dad know where I am, I thought and quickly scribbled a note on the hotel stationery that I shoved under his door before I went down. As he had been knocking back a lot of drinks, and probably more after I went to bed, I guessed he was snoring his head off. Just in case I got that wrong, I poked my head around the restaurant door. There was no sign of him or Craig and Dawn having breakfast. *I'll go and sunbathe a bit*, I told myself after helping myself to fruit, which I took outside. There were hardly any people out there, which pleased me. It meant I could choose which of the sun loungers with the hotel's neatly folded towels on them I wanted.

It didn't take long for me to feel that the pool was beckoning me to get in. Soon it would be full of the other guests, and didn't I want to try to swim while it was more or less empty? That was all it took to make me pull off my things, jump in and start swimming lengths.

By the time Dad came out looking for me, I was hungry enough to follow him into the breakfast room. He ordered us both an English breakfast, which I ate as quickly as I could because I wanted to go back outside.

'Where's Craig and Dawn?' I asked.

'Oh, I expect they'll be down soon,' he said. 'Anyhow, let's go outside. I could do with a tan. You did put some sunscreen on, didn't you?'

'Yes,' I answered as I had, but only on my front.

Dad sat on the lounger next to mine while I plunged into the water again. 'Doing well, Amy,' he told me with a grin as I stopped to hang onto the side nearest him.

I decided then that I could do better to impress him and so I climbed up the steps to the diving board. Raising my arms in the right position, I took a deep breath and dived down. I could hear Dad shouting, 'Well done, my girl,' which made me feel so proud of myself.

The only thing that went wrong was my bright red shoulders, which were very evident by lunchtime. Mum had been the one who, because I had fair skin, carefully covered all the parts the sun could get to. I clearly hadn't managed to do that very well – I was hardly able to plaster my back with it, was I?

'Goodness!' said Dawn when she saw my glowing shoulders. 'We don't want that to blister. If you go up to your bedroom, I'll bring you some after-sun lotion.'

After knocking on my door, Dawn came in and applied the lotion as gently as she could. Almost straight away, my back and shoulders began to feel less painful.

'For the rest of the holiday, cover up until I arrive,' she instructed me. 'I'll put sunscreen on for you. Now keep a shirt on until that red fades – no one minds if you're wearing it in the pool.'

I was grateful to her for both the soothing cream and the advice. My sunburn could have got far worse had she not spotted it so soon. We went back to the pool and, for the rest of the morning, I lay in the shade of a sun umbrella. I did as she had told me and, over the next few days, I pulled on a shirt until Dawn checked that every bit of my skin that was exposed to the sun was covered with enough sun cream.

That late afternoon when the temperature was cooler, we all went to the bazaar. I had pictured it in my head as being like any English market, with different goods piled on wooden tables, but that's not what it was like at all. First stop was to load ourselves up with Turkish delight. They were the most delicious sweets I had ever had. As we strolled around, I couldn't help but munch my way through the bag.

'We'll take some boxes of it back with us. I want to give a large one to Anne, she's been so good to us, and Aunt Janet and the family,' Dad said. Despite my mouth being full of Turkish delight, I found myself smiling up at him. All the bold colours of the market made it look magical and I was dazzled by the exotic stalls around us. As we walked further in, there were stalls with different types of clothing and beautiful hand-woven scarves in bright colours. Then there were the rugs, which unlike our plain cream one at home had amazing intricate patterns on them in the most vibrant colours. Some of them looked as though they could only go in a house with very large rooms but there were other, smaller ones, the right size for our house, that I wished we could take back. They looked so thick and luxuriant that I could imagine myself walking barefoot over the wonderful patterns.

As for all the leather goods, Dawn and I could barely take our eyes off them. 'They really are amazing and so are the prices,' she said happily. Looking at the collection of hand-bags prompted a wave of sadness and for a few moments I could not help but picture Mum standing there, trying to decide which one she would like.

Don't get tearful now, I told myself firmly as a treacherous lump became lodged in my throat.

Seeing me looking at the bags, Dad walked over – 'I think you'd better choose one of those. It's a girls' thing, handbags, isn't it?'

Dawn, who I felt had noticed that I was a little upset, pointed to a small bright pink one with a long strap – 'Don't you think that's the one for you, Amy? It would look stunning on your shoulder.' She signalled to the stallholder to let me have a closer look at it.

'So, what do you think?' she asked once I was standing in front of the mirror with the bag dangling on my shoulder.

'Yes, you're right, that's the one for me, and look how the strap also allows me to wear it across my body,' I told her enthusiastically.

Dawn then chose a couple of pretty pastel-coloured summer bags for herself. 'Can't resist them, I'm so fed up with navy, black and brown,' she said with a grin.

Dad bought me a new satchel as well, a really nice one that would be perfect for when I went to secondary school in September. That, my handbag and the Turkish delights were just some of the things we took back with us. I remember now that Dad bought a leather jacket but I can't remember whether he got himself anything else. Naturally, my memory of that time is a little blurred. It was over twenty years ago when we were on that holiday. Looking back on it now, despite my reluctance to go, I can see that it did me good. There was little there to remind me of Mum all the time. Of course, I missed her, but Dawn, Craig and Dad were with me nearly all the time and they all made sure that there would be new pictures in my head that I could talk about when we returned home.

There were day trips to various small towns, to the markets and the sea, and if we were missing lunch at the hotel, they would pack up a picnic for us. Swimming in that sea was amazing.

I can hardly believe now what the plan was for our last

night. First, we went out for dinner and they had a few drinks while I, as usual had soft ones. Once our meal, which was really delicious, was finished, Craig drew out a small street map. 'Know where it is,' he announced, 'so you three just follow me.'

'Where to?' I asked, because I had thought that we would all go back to the hotel.

'You'll see when we get there, Amy,' he told me, which obviously aroused my curiosity.

Being a child, I found it impossible to keep quiet as we walked towards wherever we were going.

'Come on, Craig, where are you taking us?' I asked when I caught up with him.

'All right, Amy, it's a small club where everyone is welcome,' he told me. Behind me, I heard Dawn giggling a little.

'We thought we would have a fun last night out,' she said, taking hold of my arm until we reached the road where the place was.

'Here we are,' Craig announced as we stood in front of a black door while he pressed the bell. I could see the tiny spy hole in the door, which made me realise that whoever was behind it wanted to know who was trying to come in. When the door opened, my face must have been a picture: a woman wearing tons of make-up and the tightest dress I had ever seen was there. She welcomed us in with a big smile and, leading the way, we followed her swaying hips as she showed us to a small circular table that was painted gold.

My eyes must have been everywhere, taking it all in. This was nothing like the only other club I had ever been to, the local working men's club. There was sultry music playing and another woman in a clingy red dress stood behind the bar polishing already-gleaming glasses. But it was the decor that made me stare. All the seats and the curtains were a rich, dark red, and the lights in the ceiling looked like little stars and shone down onto the tables tucked into corners. On the other side of the room was a small stage with a mic standing on it. There was even a tiny area in front of it where people could dance, or maybe where they could stand to take a better look at whoever was performing on the stage.

'Is there going to be a bit of a show?' I asked Craig.

'Something like that,' he whispered back with a grin.

Our drinks were brought over. Another alcohol-free cocktail for me and red wine for the adults. A dish with olives, nuts and small cheesy biscuits was also placed on the little table. I could hear the bell ringing periodically and, each time, a few more people came in. Up went the volume of the music. Another round of drinks later, a short, rather overweight man wearing a black velvet jacket and a red bow tie came onto the stage.

He spoke first in his own language and then in heavily accented English to announce who was coming onto the stage. 'Aylin,' he called her but, as she stepped onto the stage, I was pretty sure she was a beautiful boy, not a girl – Christmas pantos back home had taught me a few things!

She was tall and slender with long black hair and, with the light shining on it, it was so glossy that I was convinced it was a wig. I wondered what she would look like without it, but I just loved the floaty sliver dress she was wearing.

She stood in front of the mic and with great emotion sang some songs I had never heard of, which didn't stop me swaying to the music a little as well. Her voice really got to me. The finale was 'Lili Marlene'. No, I had never heard of that either, but Dawn told me it was a soldiers' love song from the war.

When the applause finished, she strutted over to our table in her skintight dress and heels.

'Hello,' she said in the highest-pitched tone she could manage.

No doubt, I decided, this was a man. I thought she looked like a princess and so I told her so.

'And you look like a pretty little one too,' she said, delighted.

It was her, the dress and the red and gold decor that formed a picture in my head which has stayed with me right up until now.

8

Having to pack my suitcase before I went down to breakfast on the last day made me feel quite sad. Turkey had become a place where I could escape from my grief. A lot of that had to do with Craig and Dawn's company. Things had been difficult between Dad and I since that awful scene in the hospital. It was they who had helped make our holiday more cheerful than I would ever have believed it could be. I wasn't looking forward to saying goodbye to them at all. If only they lived near us, but they were in the south of England and we were in the north so I didn't think I was likely to ever see them again. Maybe the odd Christmas card would drop on our mat a few times before they forgot about us. I remembered Mum talking about people we had met on previous holidays and how we had all swapped addresses, but then we never heard from them again – 'Holiday friends' she had called them.

Let's have a last swim before Dad gets up, I told myself as I pulled on my swimsuit and rushed down to the pool.

I must have spent about fifteen minutes swimming breast-stroke as fast as I could, pounding up and down repeatedly. That burst of exercise made me feel refreshed. Getting out, I shook myself like dogs do and then, wrapping myself in a towel, I went back to my room to get dressed for the journey home.

Jeans and a T-shirt with a jumper in my hand luggage just in case was the best option I decided, as Dad had said it would be quite cool when we got off that plane. I dried my hair then pulled it back into a ponytail. Just as I had finished getting ready, he knocked on the door.

'Time for breakfast, Amy.'

As if the rumbling in my stomach wasn't already telling me that, I thought grumpily.

We left our cases outside our doors and went downstairs. Craig and Dawn joined us almost straight away and, once we had finished eating, we went outside to where our minibus was parked to take us to the airport.

One of the staff wheeled our luggage out for us and then we all climbed in. The journey to the airport seemed faster than when we had arrived. We had the same driver who had brought us there and he helped us with finding a trolley to put our luggage on. I noticed that both Craig and Dad thanked him as they gave him a tip.

As our plane was leaving over half an hour earlier than Craig and Dawn's, we said our goodbyes once we were inside the airport. As Dad and I walked away, I knew that they would be missed.

This time, I had made sure I had a book to read on the

flight – Dad was not someone who chatted much on a journey. I can't remember now what the name of the book was, but at least I had something to occupy my mind and stop me from thinking about walking into an empty house without Mum.

The flight also seemed longer, probably because I didn't drift off to sleep as I had on the flight leaving England. The sun might have been shining when our plane landed but, without those glimpses of Turkey's azure blue sea, it failed to cheer me up. I thought we would have to get a taxi home, but once we had gone through customs I saw Joe, an old friend of Dad's who had marched with him in protest during the miners' strike, waiting for us at the airport exit.

'Hi John, I thought I'd give you a lift home, save you having to get a taxi,' he said, giving Dad a thump on the back and me a hug. 'Boy, you two look great! Plenty of sun in Turkey, was there?'

'There was indeed,' Dad said.

'And you, Amy, did you like it there?'

'Loved it,' I said, wishing I was still there.

'Well, let's get you both home. My car is parked close by.'

Joe insisted on wheeling the luggage trolley to where his dark blue saloon was parked. He opened the door at the back for me to get in and placed our luggage in the boot. As the car sped along, I could hear Dad telling him all about the holiday while I just gazed out of the window.

'She did well at her diving, didn't you, Amy? Got a lot of applause from the others round the pool.' Dad actually sounded quite proud of me as he told John that I had used the highest board and plunged in at the deep end of the pool.

'I think I did,' I replied as a picture came into my head of that sparkling pool with its three levels of diving boards.

As we got closer and closer to home, I could already feel the depression sneaking back on me – I was dreading going into the house. When John pulled up in front of it, I could feel the silence wrapping itself around me as I followed the two men inside. If it was all three of us as well as John who had just walked in, it would have been so different. I could almost hear Mum's voice as we brought in the luggage, the sound of her feet walking straight into the kitchen to put the kettle on. This time it was me who did that, though neither Dad nor John was interested in a hot drink. Without Mum being there, Dad pulled out a couple of beers from the fridge – something he just wouldn't have done before within minutes of us returning from a holiday; Mum would have had something to say about that.

'Cheers, mate, and thanks,' said Dad as he took a long swig from the bottle (Mum would have insisted they use glasses).

'And cheers to you both. Your tea all right, Amy?'

'Yes,' I muttered as I perched on the high wooden stool next to the breakfast bar.

There was more conversation about our holiday floating around me and I had little to add other than to nod when Dad asked me to confirm how great it all was. I could hear him saying that he'd taken some good photos and was going to get a few of them enlarged – 'I'll get some of them framed and hang them up in the sitting room. Good idea, don't you think, Amy?'

The answer that nearly shot out of my mouth was a firm

'no'. I didn't want pictures of a holiday without Mum in them, but that little voice in my head told me to say nothing. So, after taking a deep breath, I sensibly managed a smile and agreed with him.

More beer came out of the fridge and, knowing these would not be the last ones, I made an excuse that I wanted to unpack and went upstairs to my room. I could hear the men's laughter getting louder and louder. Like Mum, I didn't like seeing my father drunk because he was unpredictable then.

I heard John leaving quite a while later. Clearly, he did not have a problem driving when he was over the limit. I just hoped that Dad wouldn't continue drinking then.

It must have been about an hour later that the doorbell rang.

I hope that's not John back with more booze, I said to myself as I went down to see who it was. To my relief, it was not him on our doorstep but Anne, holding a large carrier bag.

'I brought you and your dad some food,' she said and then told me how good I looked as she walked through to the kitchen.

Luckily, my appetite had come back on the holiday. My mouth watered as I watched her unpack a whole roast chicken, some potatoes that she told me only needed heating up in the microwave and another container with a healthy-looking salad in it.

'Thought that would last you until tomorrow and then your dad can go shopping,' she said, while I put the kettle back on. 'I see you found the milk I got in for you. Did you find the chocolate biscuits I left in the tin?'

The sound of the doorbell ringing and our chatter must have woken Dad. I had seen him dozing in front of the television and, not knowing who was at the door, I had closed it quietly. He came into the kitchen and gave Anne a hug, especially after seeing what she had brought over for us.

'Thank you, Anne. We've got a little something for you from our holiday,' he said and out he went into the hall, where his case was still standing, and pulled out the large box of Turkish delight.

I prayed she couldn't smell the drink on his breath but, if she did, nothing was said. She just invited me to spend the following day with her and the children – 'You can tell them all about your holiday, can't you? You can have lunch with us and then I'll bring you back sometime in the afternoon.'

'That's nice of you, Anne. I don't want Amy getting bored just being with me,' said Dad.

I guessed that, without me under his feet, he felt free to meet up with some of his friends again.

'That's great, Anne, thank you,' was my answer.

After she left, we tucked into the food she had brought. Then we watched a bit of TV before I took myself up to bed as Dad poured himself a whisky from the litre bottle that he had bought at the Duty Free.

The next morning, I got ready to walk over to Anne's. I could hear Dad snoring when I walked past his bedroom to go downstairs. He must have been full of beer and whisky, I thought, as I tipped some breakfast cereal into a bowl, poured some milk over it and gulped it down.

At least I'll have company at Anne's, I thought.

And make sure you look cheerful, said that annoying little voice in my head.

I never told Anne that Dad was asleep when I left or that he had carried on drinking, though having been a friend, she most probably knew about all the problems Mum was having with him, especially over his drinking. Not that she would ever have said anything to me.

Being at Anne's home was so relaxing. I did talk about the holiday, but I left out the details of our last evening – I knew it wasn't necessarily appropriate for a girl of my age and I didn't think Anne would approve. Her sons were a little younger than me, which didn't stop them asking quite a few questions about what we had done there. After I had exhausted my holiday tales, we all went out into the garden and had some fun playing with a ball.

So what was the evening like when I returned home? Even though I had eaten a big lunch, I joined Dad in the kitchen and had some of Anne's chicken. After Dad had finished, he said he was going to watch the football and so he went into the sitting room with a six-pack of beer. He drank one beer after the other until I took myself off to bed.

I now knew that this was what my life with him was going to be like.

9

There was only a week left before I was due to begin a new school year. I felt a little nervous because, as I had turned eleven before our holiday, I would now be at the senior school. It was just a short bus trip from our home, but what with our holiday and also my depression after Mum's death, I had not seen much of anyone from school during the holidays. That meant I wasn't sure who else from our village might be on that morning's bus as well. Most probably very few, as most mothers would be taking their children to the first day at their new school.

Mum would have done the same, but Dad never even suggested it. 'You know where the bus stop is' was the only remark he made on the subject when I reminded him that I was changing schools. Another thing was playing on my mind was that I wasn't happy about having to wear the new uniform. I can't say I liked it very much. Again, it was Anne who had taken me to the shops to help me buy everything I needed.

Black blazer, black trousers or a black skirt. At least we could wear white shirts, but not pretty ones – they had to have the right collar so we could wear ties. And ties were not something I wanted to wear; besides, I had no idea how to tie them.

'Dad, can you show me how to put a tie on?' It was one of the few times I asked him for help. Not that he often wore a tie himself – in his line of work it was only for special occasions.

'No problem,' he answered with a grin, 'not that I like wearing them either.'

That lesson of tying it the right way was a bit of fun between us anyhow and, after a few tries, I got it right. He was pleased with that but not with the slouch socks – fashionable then – that I had chosen.

'They look dreadful, as though they're sliding down your legs,' he observed.

'But they're meant to be like this, Dad – everyone's wearing them,' I insisted.

'Oh, all right, seems it's a good name for them. As long as the teachers don't object. At least the rest of your uniform is smart.'

That was the end of that conversation as he looked again at my socks, shook his head in disbelief and opened the fridge for a beer.

Back then, I was still the kind of girl most people would have described as a well-mannered child. I seldom argued with anyone and did as I was told. Dad's friends, my aunts and Anne considered me to be a nice young girl. If Mum had lived, I have no doubt that I would have got through my teenage years with them still thinking that. Sadly, that nice child was not far off changing to one who eventually made those who had cared for her have a completely different opinion.

The beginning of the change in me started not long after I moved to my senior school. It just took one boy's insult to trigger what was the good child in me to evaporate.

10

I had begun sorting out what I needed for school over the weekend before the new academic year started but I couldn't stop worrying about what it was going to be like there. Would the teachers, who would have been told everything about my recent family tragedy, send me the glances of pity which I had seen all too often from other people? Before junior school broke up, I could almost hear my schoolteachers talking about me. I had seen their looks of concern when they knew my mother was in hospital so gravely ill.

To be fair, after they had been informed that she had died, they did their best to look out for me. Still all those glances that so often came in my direction from people who knew about her death made me cringe. Maybe what people don't understand is that too much sympathy is a constant reminder of the loss of the person who was loved so deeply. I just didn't want to be treated any differently to the other pupils in my class. While I had known all the teachers at my junior school, I hadn't met any of the ones at the new one. It was the not knowing anything about them and how they might react when I walked into the classroom that was niggling away at me. The last thing I wanted was any more pity.

I had heard so many remarks about me after Mum died. Even once when I was on holiday, trying my hardest to put everything behind me. I had gone into the reception area to see if Dad was about when I heard the hotel manager talking to Dawn and Craig about me – 'Poor little girl, so young to have lost her mother. It must be so awful for her,' he was saying.

On hearing this, I scuttled away as fast as I could. I don't know if I was seen and, if I had been, they were sensible enough not to say anything to me. I know now that it wasn't Craig and Dawn who had told them because of course the manager would have known because Dad would have had to take Mum's name off the booking, as well as explain the reason why. No wonder the staff had been so helpful to us, and why Dawn and Craig had been so kind to me.

The other remarks I had overheard before the holiday have stuck in my mind right up until now. I know I was not meant to hear them, but I did. Some came from Mum's nurses, others from Anne's neighbours when they whispered to her on the doorstep. Then there were a few who came into Anne's house for a cup of tea and stopped talking when I entered the room. I just couldn't bear any more of it. Mostly it upset me so badly, I wanted to sit in a room on my own and cry. Even at that age, I hated anyone seeing tears in my eyes. Ever since I had cried at the funeral, I had done my best to hide my grief. There were so many questions I had over Mum being in hospital, her death and what had caused it. I know they were difficult ones for the adults to answer. They must have understood that the reason I wanted to know was that I was still trying to make sense of her sudden death and because I missed her so much.

I shall never ever forget that visit to the hospital, any more than I can Dad's reaction to Mum recognising me but not him. And why had she been so angry with him as he stood next to me?

I suppose I was oversensitive at that time, but surely that's understandable. When I bumped into classmates who I had never been that friendly with, they were nice enough to me and I put it down to them hearing about Mum. Had their parents told them to be kind to me? Did they stop and reflect how they might be feeling if their parent had just died suddenly? Did they pity me? I asked myself these questions every time it happened.

Now my adult self thinks it was just that they were actually just nice people. We might not have been close friends, simply because we didn't have much in common, but that was hardly a reason for them not to be kind.

Come on, Amy, I told myself before the term began, *most of your classmates are all right, apart from a boy called Ron.* He'd been in my class at primary school and was lanky with mousey hair, a swaggering walk and a mouth that always seemed twisted into an unpleasant smirk.

It was not so much the smirk that bothered me, it was his eyes. Pale grey ones that barely blinked when he stared at me, as he did with a few of the other girls. I could tell by his smirk that he enjoyed making us feel uneasy. I know that he made some of us feel really scared of him and we did our best to avoid him. I, on the other hand, one time, had met his gaze and gave him a blank look before I turned and walked slowly away. That irritated him no end apparently, or so I was told – 'He really glared at your back and muttered something like "stuck-up bitch",' one of the girls told me.

'I don't care,' I said because it pleased me that I was getting to him. Not that it stopped me from keeping as far away from him as possible.

'He's so creepy,' was the description a friend of mine – Maddy – had used and a few others who heard her agreed, advising, 'It's best to keep away from him. There's something seriously wrong with that boy.'

'He's horrid and he smells. A fox was in our shed and he smells just like that,' said another and we giggled.

A few more similar remarks began coming from the other girls. Not that we wanted him to hear us because, considering his age, his tongue was a viciously sharp and an insulting one too. However, when my thoughts turned to my senior school and what I needed for it, Ron really didn't come into my mind and I had no idea whether he would also be transferring to the new school. Had I thought about it, I'm sure that it would have added to my sense of apprehension.

Every other year when the holidays were coming to an end, I looked forward to going back to school and catching up with some of my classmates. This time I didn't feel that way. I just hoped all the talk would be about the holidays, but I really didn't want to hear a word about Mum. I suppose, to them, it was old news as she had died five months before but to me it was as if it were yesterday. My whole life was divided into with Mum and without Mum. Maybe if she had been diagnosed with a terminal illness and her death had come after months of suffering, I might have managed better but it was all just so sudden.

The day I took myself off to my new school, I tried to look as nonchalant as I could. It was surprising when we all met up in the new playground. Had my fellow pupils' parents told them to be tactful about what they said to me? Maybe, or had time just moved on and to them, I was just the kid without a mother? They certainly managed not to ask the wrong questions.

I soon found that chatting away about my holiday was pretty easy – after all, we had done quite a lot there. Some of my friends had gone camping with their parents in the south of England, a couple had gone to Spain, but no one had ever been to a place like Turkey. Not wanting to make them jealous, I was cautious about what I said about our luxurious hotel and the bazaar but they encouraged me to tell them more. And what girl of that age doesn't want to hear about shopping?

By the end of the first day, my worries about the new school had disappeared – in fact, I felt quite settled. The teachers were friendly, nothing difficult was said to me that I didn't want to hear and I was able to sit next to Maddy. Over the next few days, I was invited to her house so we could work on our homework together. That invitation was gratefully accepted. Anne's children would be wanting me to play with them and I hated going back to an empty house and spending most of the evening alone because Dad was out drinking after work.

By the end of the first week, I told myself that I had been silly to have worried so much about changing school. Well, I was hardly able to see into the future, was I? If I had, I might have seen that a lot was going to change for me the following Friday when a ball of grief slammed into me. I still only have a partial memory of it and it was Anne who tried to fill in the gaps afterwards. She explained what had happened and why it had affected me so much.

'It was that awful boy, wasn't it?' I said dolefully. 'The one who has always been rude to me. He hates me and keeps calling me a spoilt little bitch and saying I thought I was better than everyone.'

'Yes, it was him – Ron, you said his name is.' She asked me what I could remember and I told her that the beginning of the day was clear in my head. As I did every school day, I got myself ready, made sure my hair was neatly brushed and that my clothes were freshly ironed. Dad now used a laundry service but, as things got worse, he sometimes forgot to collect it unless I reminded him.

It was on our mid-morning break when a classmate who I didn't know very well came up and asked me what Turkey was like – 'My mother told me we might go next year.'

'Oh, you'll love it. It's so beautiful. Miles of white sand and you should see the bazaars! Tell your mum that leather handbags and coats are really cheap there and the food is fantastic. The people are so friendly as well,' I said.

As I thought of how the conversation had developed, some of the memories of what happened came back to me. I remember that, when I was talking to the girl, I heard a boy's voice behind me saying, 'There she goes, boasting again.' Spinning around, I saw Ron standing just a couple of feet away. I might have forgotten how nasty he could be, but I had also felt relieved that we were not in the same class. *He's trying to annoy me again, just ignore him*, I told myself and, with my head held high, I began walking away from him. This time my lack of a reaction must have annoyed him so much that his hand landed on my back and he shoved me forward. That was enough to make me turn round and glare at him.

I received a mocking smirk back that just infuriated me. If only I had clenched my hands and walked away – but I didn't. Instead, I pulled my shoulders back and looked straight into his face as I snapped angrily, 'Will you just leave me alone? I think you're awful and I bet everyone else does as well.'

There was silence around me then, all eyes must have been fixed on us. I heard Maddy whispering, 'Amy, come on, let's go,' but it was too late, he was already fired up.

'What do you think you're saying? You spoilt little bitch! You still think you're better than us, but I've got something you haven't and never will.'

And that's when he really let rip and I froze.

'I've got a mum, not a dead one with no brain. Do you hear me? Your mum was burnt into little pieces and the wind blew them away. My mum's still here and so is her brain. You hear me?'

That was when that ball of sadness shot forward and knocked

me flying. Apparently, I flew at him, my fingers stretched out, clawing at his face. I know I was screaming and that he was shouting at me to stop. I heard another voice saying my name in a calm but firm voice; it must have been one of the teachers. I have a vague recollection of her arm going round me and pulling me away from him. The rest is blank.

Anne told me that the teacher had asked the others, 'Whatever has happened here?' 'Several pupils told her what he had said about your mother.' What she didn't tell me was that one of the teachers had told Dad that my actions had frightened all the pupils near me – I must have looked completely crazy to them.

'I suppose my screaming didn't stop then because my throat was still sore?'

'Yes, you did for quite a while, but then it turned into sobs.'

'What happened then?'

'Another teacher came, one of the girls was sent to get the head and then everyone except the boy was told to go into their classroom.'

'What happened to him?'

'I don't know, except for what your dad told me. The boy had to sit outside the head teacher's office for a while after the nurse had checked the scratches on his face and his parents were called into the school later. I heard that it took a while for you to calm down, not that anything could stop your sobbing. You were picked up by one of the male teachers and carried into a room where there was a couch. He laid you down on it. It was the head who sat by you after she told the teachers to go back to their classes.'

'I must have almost passed out for a while, Anne. I can remember the head holding my hand and helping me sit up then asking if I was feeling a little better. I was so confused when I looked round the unfamiliar room that I don't think I replied. I remember her giving me a hot sugary drink to sip and telling me that a doctor was coming to see me. She also said that I needn't worry about getting home because she had spoken to Dad and he was coming to take me back.

'I don't know how long it took for the doctor to arrive – I think I must have drifted off a little. I can't picture what she looked like, although I do remember it was a woman, but all but I can remember was one sentence that stuck in my mind: "Sometimes the shock of a death doesn't come straight away," she told me. "It clearly came to you today and that's more normal than you must be thinking."

'That made me feel a little better.

'I wonder now if she gave me a sedative. It's all so muddled, Anne. Dad must have come and taken me home, but I can't remember that or how I got into bed with my pyjamas on.'

'I went over and helped him there,' Anne explained with a smile.

Even now there are things that happened that day of which I have no memory. Or maybe I don't want to bring it all back. But I can say that there was lasting harm done to me. I've never been able to forget those cruel words Ron spewed out at me. I knew then, and I know now, that much of it was the truth – a truth that I had tried to block from my mind. The picture of Mum's happy face when we went to Cleethorpes was the one I had wanted to keep in my head. It was Ron's words that changed that picture forever to the one of her in hospital, wired up to machines and her face distorted with anger when she didn't recognise Dad. Try as I might to dislodge it and wipe it from my memory, it is still fixed in my mind right up to today.

11

I was off school for at least two or three weeks after the trauma of that day. Nobody put a name to what was wrong with me then, now I would say it was a breakdown. Most of what happened during those weeks has remained a blur. I can remember there was someone, a woman who came to the house at least once or twice a week, not just to talk to me but to get me to tell her about my feelings. I know it made me cry quite a bit. Dad continued going out to work, and going out with his mates, leaving me at home alone, and so Anne came over every day while her children were at school.

'I can see you're starting to feel better,' she told me when, for the first time in what seemed like weeks, I decided to get dressed instead of sitting up in my bed or coming downstairs for a while in my dressing gown.

It was me who made up my mind that it was time for me to go back to school.

'Are you sure you're ready for it? Your teachers could send

you some more work to do at home for a little while longer,' Anne suggested.

'That wouldn't be enough,' I told her. 'I would get really behind in my classes and I don't want that. Today's Wednesday, isn't it?'

'Yes, it is.'

'So, I was thinking that I will go in on Monday.'

She smiled at that and gave me a hug. 'Good for you, dear,' she said. But I felt she was not as pleased as she pretended to be.

Dad, on the other hand was much happier about the whole thing. 'Heard you're going back to school on Monday,' he said and I could see that he was looking relieved. He surprised me a little with his next remark: 'You've only been with Anne and me for quite a long time – well, apart from the therapist, that is. I think it would be a good idea if you came out with me on Friday for the family night at the club. Are you up to that?'

I felt a little nervous at the suggestion, but he was right, I needed to get used to being in a busy place and seeing other people.

'Yes, Dad, I'll go with you,' I said.

'Good for you,' he told me and, for once, he patted me on my back.

Although a lot of my memories are jumbled up, which makes it sometimes difficult to put them in order, that particular evening is clear to me. Even better, the couple of days that preceded it are too.

'They're having karaoke this week and you've got a good

voice. I've told them that and they're looking forward to seeing you give it a go so you choose what you want to sing,' Dad said.

My legs started shaking. I had thought the evening would involve just sitting there and talking to the people who came over. Singing on the little stage in the club in front of a room full of strangers was quite another thing. What would happen if I didn't do well? Would they laugh at me? My mind was full of fear and self-doubt. As though Dad could read my mind, he said, 'Now don't you let me down, Amy. You sort out something pretty to wear. You could go through Mum's music collection and choose something in it to sing, couldn't you?'

'Yes, I could,' I replied, still hesitantly. Hadn't Mum sung there more than once and hadn't everyone loved her voice? But it was not just her voice but the songs she had chosen.

'All right, Dad,' was about all I could say, still terrified at the thought.

I thought about the songs I knew – there weren't many, but there was one that Mum had sung at the club before. She was such a big fan of the Carpenters and I suddenly remembered her singing one of their greatest hits, 'Top of the World'. She often sung it around the house too when she was happy. And I suddenly wanted to sing her favourite song and get it right, just for her.

I had a search through the CDs and, not finding it, I went through some of the cassettes my parents had bought way back when. There was the faded cassette of *Carpenters – The Singles*. When I found it, I played and played it until the words were drummed into my head.

Dad actually cooked us breakfast that Friday morning before Anne arrived. When she came into the kitchen, she looked pleased to see us finishing it together.

'You and your family coming to the club tonight, Anne? Amy here's going to sing.'

'Well then, we'd better make sure we do,' she said with a smile.

'I'm looking forward to tonight, love,' he told me and he actually took my hand and squeezed it.

I hope Anne didn't get too fed up of hearing that song being played more than a few times during the day. At least by the afternoon when she left, I was pretty sure that I knew all the words. I had a bubble bath, washed my hair and chose a dress that I knew Dad liked – it was the deep blue one with a flared skirt that I had worn on our holiday. My hair was blow-dried and hung loose. When I heard him coming through the door, I went downstairs. On seeing me, he smiled – which he didn't do too often – and told me I looked nice. He had brought a Chinese takeaway with him, which we ate together before he drove us to the club.

I was very nervous about whether I would remember all the words. Never having done karaoke, I had no idea that all the words would come up on the screen for me to read. Had I known that, I might have felt a bit more confident.

When we reached the club and walked in, there were lots of smiles and friendly greetings. We sat at the same table where, not so long ago, the three of us had often sat. As people came over to chat to us, Dad told them that I was going to sing, which caused more smiles to come in my direction.

A couple of people went up to the stage and sang. After a few songs, I heard the voice of the man with the karaoke machine calling out my name: 'Amy, you're up next. Give her a clap, everyone.' The noise of all that clapping seemed pretty loud to me.

A hand reached out to help me up onto the stage and the mic was placed in my hand. I pictured my mother then and almost heard her voice in my head when she sang there. I closed my eyes, for I didn't need the screen, did I? As I sang the first notes, I could have heard a pin drop. When the last note left my lips, the applause that I received was thunderous. My eyes flickered open and I glanced over in Dad's direction. I swear that just for a moment, I saw Mum standing there right next to him, smiling up at me. As I looked in total disbelief, it was as though a mist enveloped her and, with only another blink of my eyes, she disappeared. Whatever you think, I'm not exaggerating or making this up, I swear that she had been there watching me. I remember it so well and how I wanted to call out for her to stay, but common sense stopped me.

When I was back at the table, people came over to me, saying that I had a voice so like my mother's. Some of them asked me to sing again, but I just couldn't bring myself to do it.

'Another night maybe, but my throat's a bit sore,' was my excuse.

I noticed that Dad did not ask me to sing again.

There were a few other Friday nights when he took me with him. Saturdays were the days I was left in the house on my own. There were always excuses such as he had to meet a pal or there was a union meeting. Like Mum experienced, there were times when I heard the sound of the car that had brought him home driving off as he walked in on unsteady feet.

12

What does a lonely young girl do to enable her to express her feelings? She gets a diary and, on its pages, she can tell it everything. When I read through it after all the years that have passed, I can see my younger self and feel her unhappiness and I find myself sliding back in time and stepping into her shoes. I watch her taking those disastrous steps which took her down a dangerous path and mixing with the wrong people; people who nearly destroyed her. The grammar in that diary was hardly correct, nor were some of words spelt correctly, and on occasions even incorrect words were used, so a little prudent editing was needed here before I felt able to share it with you!

Since that breakdown where I screamed and sobbed in front of so many pupils who barely knew me, everything has changed. The ones who had been friendly before that scene now try to avoid me. I know I'm getting fatter, for isn't food meant to be a comfort? Must be all those takeaways that I eat on my own when Dad has left the money on the kitchen table for me to order in. They're big enough for two, but I never leave any of it, do I? It's them and you too, diary, who are the only things to ease my pain. You're my best friend now. It's the first time since I started at secondary school that I feel as if I have one. I think it was hearing the words 'brain dead' going through my head again and again that started my screaming. Those who had once been friendly have slipped away from me, probably because I scared them so much.

Now I'm getting podgy, which is another thing that depresses me. They've nicknamed me Teletubby and it causes a lot of laughing especially from the ones I hadn't got on with before. They snigger when they pass me on our breaks and give me sly looks as they nudge each other, saying, 'Move over, here comes the Teletubby.' It's as though all the sympathy they had for me because of Mum has left them.

It seems that the months are just sliding away and I get more miserable. Everyone told me my grieving would get less with time, but it doesn't. Dad hardly bothers with me. He's not mentioned us going on another summer holiday. I won't ask about it. I don't want to hear any more of his excuses. Like why he has to go out most nights. I can tell he's doesn't want to spend time with me. I suppose he did try for a while, but that's all gone out the window now. I hate going home to an empty house, it makes me feel so lonely. It was all so different when Mum was there. The dishwasher would be rumbling or the kettle whistling when I came in, the air would be fragrant with cooking smells and her voice always calling out to me as I opened the front door. When I think of how it was then, how I'd sit down in the kitchen with her, munch a biscuit and drink the tea she made. I'd tell her about my day and she would tell me about her's. I'd better stop writing this as I can feel tears already in the back of my throat. Don't want them dropping all over you, do I?

There's another thing that's upsetting me: I keep asking myself where are my aunts and uncles and where are all Mum's friends, the ones who were so often knocking on our door and dropping off casseroles? Now there's only Anne who comes to see me. Has everyone forgotten that I'm still alive, even if Mum is dead?

And why won't Aunt Janet stay with us when she visits our town? Instead, she goes and stays with other friends who live nearby. It must be something to do with me. But I miss her as well. When Mum was still here, she was the sister closest to her and the one I loved the most. They were always on the phone chatting away. Then the words I wanted to hear came, 'Yes, we're free next weekend,' Mum would say before winking at me, 'Amy and I are looking forward to you coming already!' I was as delighted as Mum when I knew she was going to stay with us for a long weekend.

Oh, I know, she still does some of right things when

she's in town, like taking me out to a café for tea, or if the cinema has a suitable film for my age group. But that's not the same, is it? Is she just doing her duty? I wish she would stay with us – I would like so much just to come down the stairs in the morning and be able to sit and chat while we had breakfast. If Dad can be bothered, he just puts it on the table for me and picks up the newspaper. But even more important is the thought of leaving school, knowing she would be here. The house would feel like a home again.

13

Now, over twenty years later, my adult self understands my aunt's reasons for not wanting to come and stay in our house. She simply did not approve of Dad. Her local friends had told her a few things about him, such as how, in the club and bars, he flashed money about. Where did that money come from? I know now that it came from Mum's life insurance. Which meant that, as well as no longer having to pay the mortgage, a six-figure sum had gone into his bank account. A lot of money now, let alone in the 1990s.

Of course, I didn't have any idea about that until I was quite a few years older. Nor was I aware of the verbal insults he abused Janet with. That side of Dad was not something I had ever seen, especially when Mum was alive. Though judging from some of the rows I had heard, she, too, saw something of his other side.

The next part of my younger self's life began the day I went and visited Jacqui Turner, the woman that the neighbours called the local drunk. But I and others thought there was more to her than that.

I'm forcing my mind back over a couple of decades to work out just how it was that I met her. I know the place she lived in changed not only my life, but me as well. From my diary, I can see that I hadn't turned twelve when I first met her. I can also understand why my younger self felt happy to have company there and not take any notice of certain things that happened in that house.

Before I met Jacqui and all the people who visited her, I was still innocent enough not to know anything about drugs or underage drinking. When I sat around with some of her visitors who were only a little older than me, I assumed that it was cider they were drinking. At the time, I believed we were all just having fun.

How did my downfall begin? In reality, it started the day I went to Jacqui 's house – that answer was clear to me as I flicked through another one of my diaries. It has not been easy for me to read them, but I've persevered so that I'm able to dig into those memories and bring them alive again in my mind's eye.

I'm in the school toilet, looking at myself in the mirror, and it's only my reflection that is there with me. No one else is in there and I must have spoken out my thoughts aloud. 'I don't want to go home,' I am saying to it, 'I hate walking in now that Mum's not there. It's not a home, it's where I live.' I feel tears running down my face and as I lift my hand to wipe them away, I hear a voice behind me saying, 'I know why you're sad, Amy, but you're brave, aren't you?' I feel an arm coming around my shoulder and a hand soothingly brushes back tendrils of hair clinging to the tears on my cheeks.

In the mirror, I can see the face of a girl, who as she is a couple of years older than me, was in a different class. She's tall and slim with a mane of thick blonde hair and like most pupils, I've noticed her in the playground. I know her name, it's Donna – I had heard her friends calling out to her more than once but neither of us had ever spoken to each other before today.

'I heard what you were saying to yourself, Amy. That you hate going back to an empty house, I can understand that. Look, there's a few of us going to a friend of mine's place. She welcomes everyone who goes there and we all like to have somewhere warm to go, where we can hang out after school. So, would you like to come with me there?'

I don't have to think about it and quickly say yes as I turn my head and smile gratefully at her. I don't tell her that Dad hardly ever comes home straight from work or that he seldom cooks a meal for us. Instead, he leaves me money and takeaway menus out so I can order what I like but what I really want is more than food, it's someone to talk to.

I know she's offering to take me there because she saw me crying and feels sorry for me but she's nice enough not to show it. Her arm stays round me as we walk out of the toilets and I see a couple of her friends waiting outside for her.

'I've invited Amy here to join us,' is all she says to them and thankfully not one of them asks why. Most probably, by the way they all give me warm friendly smiles, they already know the reason Donna is bringing me with them.

'You're going to have some fun with us,' says one.

'That's right,' says another, which makes me feel I'm welcome in their company.

While strolling along beside Donna, she tells me a little about the woman whose house we are on the way to.

'She has two children,' Donna is saying. 'Well, her young daughter is still a child, she's only about six, but her son Dave is well into his teens. Anyhow, Dave has his own friends, so we don't see him much. Jacqui let him turn his bedroom into a sort of a bedsit and he and his friends spend time up there, means he doesn't mind us. You will like Jacqui's, really great music system. She's happy to have her house full with a crowd from our school and she lets us choose what music we want to listen to.

'Mind you when you meet her, she might seem odd, but she's fun. Seems she doesn't want anyone around who's the same age as her. Must be because we make her feel young, even though she's not.'

'Well, I guessed that she wasn't if her son's older than me,' I say, grinning a little.

Donna points to one of the big modern houses in the estate we have just walked into and tells me we're here.

From the number of windows I see, I guess there's at least three bedrooms there. The paintwork on the house still looked fresh and new, which is more than I can say for the garden. I can feel my eyes widening at the state it's in. Not a flower nor a shrub in sight, just weeds and litter falling out of an overflowing dustbin.

Seeing my expression, Donna lets out a laugh. 'That reminds me, I think I forgot to tell you that she's probably a bit pissed by now. She likes her drink all right. Don't know if she even pours tea or coffee into a cup when she wakes up, I've only ever seen a glass in her hand.'

I just shrug my shoulders as nonchalantly as I can, though what Donna has just told me doesn't bother me a scrap. After all, I know Dad and his friends drink, even though at that time I'd never met a woman who gets tipsy in the daytime.

Still, I'm surprised when Donna, with her friends bunched up behind us, just pushes open the door without knocking first. She pulls me in with her and calls out to the woman lying on the settee: 'Hi Jacqui, I've brought a new friend with us today.'

Hearing her, Jacqui puts the glass she's holding down on the small table in front of her and walks over to me. Her eyes narrow a little as she peers into my face and then she smiles.

'So, what's your name, dear?'

'Amy.'

'Mmm, you're a pretty little thing.'

As I had put on weight from eating too many take-aways, she's the first person to pay me a compliment in quite a while.

'How old are you, Amy?' she asks and I tell her that I'm nearly twelve.

'Thought that's the age you are,' she says and her head turns towards Donna. 'You had better give her lemonade, there's some in the fridge.' I don't realise it then but in her own way, she's telling Donna not to give me alcohol. I'm too busy feeling puzzled by her voice because it's a posh one, but her clothes certainly aren't. With her long dark hair, which is streaked with grey and needs a good brush, she looks a real mess. As for her clothes, she's wearing a long, almost ankle-length, grubby denim skirt and a bright red top with stains down the front. Despite the web of wrinkles around her eyes and the deeper lines across her forehead, there's such a youthful air about her which makes me smile up at her and I know that I already like her.

I can't help looking all around me and I can see that the house is pretty messy. Apart from the haze of cig-arette smoke floating around, there's an atmosphere that makes me feel comfortable. It's a long wide room with loads of cushions on the floor for us to sit on and there's a large, open-plan kitchen at the end of it.

Minutes later, I hear the door opening and a sandy-haired boy with a dimple in his chin walks in. I see his eyes darting around the room without smiling at even one of us.

'See you're here again,' he says to Donna, without even looking in my direction.

'Hello, Dave,' she replies only to receive an unfriendly smile as he walks across the room to the kitchen. Without saying another word, he takes something from the fridge and slides it into his pocket.

When I read that part of my diary now, I have a shrewd idea of what it was Dave put in his pocket. Almost certainly heroin or another type of drug. Thankfully, my eleven-year-old self had no idea then.

A couple of minutes later, I hear the door opening again. This time another older boy wearing a black tracksuit appears. I recognise him from school – he is the one lots of the girls keep talking hopefully about. He gives us a friendly smile, says hello to Jacqui and then he and Dave take themselves off upstairs.

Donna tells me that Dave is Jacqui's son and the other boy is Pete, his closest friend. He seems much nicer and friendlier.

In my early diaries, there is no mention that my younger self was warned about getting close to those young men, who were both drug addicts and dealers. That was not all they were up to either. As I flick through the handwritten pages, I'm amazed at my naivety and can't find any remarks about my younger self being warned of the dangers of taking drugs. Or maybe Donna and her friends, who I had only seen getting

smashed on cider, didn't know either. A later diary, which I
will come to soon, makes me remember how I did find out,
but I believed by then that it was too late to walk away.

14

I can remember so clearly now what my visits to Jacqui were like. As I read my diary, everything comes flooding back to me and makes me full of guilt.

I am happier than I have been since I returned to school after my attacking Ron. I find being at Jacqui's relaxing and I'm not lonely anymore. It's so good to have company after school, even if I'm still unpopular with the others in my class. I'm not bothered at all that everyone at Jacqui's is older than me. They don't seem to mind either, they nearly always include me in their chatter although there are things I can't quite follow.

Today, I met Jacqui's young daughter, Sophia. She's so sweet, I really like her. A little brown-haired child who's only six, she sits as close to Jacqui as she can. There's something about her that makes me feel she needs looking after. I know I like Jacqui a lot, but I don't think she's a very good mother. That disappoints

me a little because I know how important a mother's
love is, but I can tell she loves her daughter.

Had I known about all the drug-users' needles and syringes
in the kitchen drawers and the supplies in the fridge, I might
have thought differently. But thank goodness I hadn't seen
them, although I wouldn't have recognised what they were –
not then anyhow. Over the time I knew Jacqui, I realised that
she loved alcohol more than she did either of her offspring.

I remember how shocked I was when I saw that Jacqui
was drunk when her daughter arrived back from school.
Mum would never have allowed me to come home on my
own at that age. Like many alcoholics I came to know over
the next few years, she managed to hold her drink well, just
not well enough for her small daughter's wellbeing. What
I've learnt since then is that alcoholics are seldom big eaters,
for an empty stomach hastens the absorption of alcohol into
the bloodstream.

I had wondered how Sophia got back as her school was
some distance away. I found out that she travelled by taxi,
one that was booked twice a day to take her there and to
bring her back home. Jacqui also used childminders so that,
if she needed a break, her daughter could stay overnight
with them. As a mother myself, Jacqui's irresponsibility
shocks me, but I think I was too relieved to have company
not to question too much.

There are other things about Jacqui's house that I dislike
a little, such as the state the kitchen is in. It's the messiest

one I have ever seen with scraps of food on the floor, a pile of dirty dishes and an overflowing bin which stinks. I can imagine what Mum would say if she was here. I can almost hear her clicking her tongue in disgust and saying, 'Needs a good clean, Amy, for the child's sake.' Well, what choice did I have? I set about cleaning it up today as best I could, but there was little in the way of cleaning materials in an overflowing cupboard.

'Well, thanks, darling,' was all that Jacqui said when she saw what I had done.

It's when I look in the fridge to see if that too needs cleaning that I get a real shock. It certainly does and there's hardly any food in it except for some that smells rotten and there's also plenty of mildewed stuff that has been spilt in there and dried solid. It seems that Jacqui's idea of grocery shopping is more about ordering bottles of wine and Sophia's lemonade. The cider is stacked neatly under the table now and there's a shelf with quite a few bottles of gin. When I look in the cupboards, I see that at least there's some breakfast cereal, a few packets of biscuits and some tins of baked beans. Tucked behind them are other tins with corned beef and fish in them. So that's all Sophia gets for supper, I suppose, and what does Jacqui eat? The same, I guess. No wonder she and her daughter are stick-thin. I've made up my mind to take food over for Sophia. I order Thai or Chinese takeaways all the time. Dad doesn't care how much I eat or how much it costs. I'll just have one meal for myself from now on. After all, I've been eating too much, haven't I? I can take the second meal with me to school then I can give it to Sophia in the afternoon.

A little later in my diary, I write about Sophia's reaction:

She really loves that food, so I must keep getting it for her. With a wide smile on her face, which I hadn't seen before, she tucked in and didn't leave one grain of rice on the plate. She even had a go with the chopsticks, giggling as noodles dropped onto the kitchen table.

Another 'Thank you, darling' came my way when Jacqui saw her daughter smiling with pleasure as she ate the food I had given her.

I can picture the scene now. Sophia was a little girl who I knew needed more care and affection than she got at home. It was partly that I had taken a liking to her daughter that made me keep going to Jacqui's. I suppose, in a way, thinking about someone else instead of myself did me good. One of the things I liked doing for Sophia apart from bringing food was finding my favourite books from when I was her age. Those I took over and, once she went to bed, I would go and read to her. That seemed to amuse Jacqui, but it certainly pleased Sophia.

Being there some days without Donna made me more aware of Jacqui's son Dave and the reasons why I disliked him. One of the first thing I noticed was that he never seemed to talk to his little sister, not even saying hello to her when he came into the house. In fact, it looked as if he was pretending that he hadn't even seen her. I saw the hurt in her eyes when she looked up at him hopefully. That was enough to make me dislike him. The only thing I knew about what might have made Dave reject his little sister was that her father was not the same one as his. Jacqui and Dave had been living with a man when she became pregnant with Sophia. That led to rows, as had her drinking, especially when she was pregnant with his child. That's about all I knew, although it puzzled me why Dave had chosen to live with his mother and not his father. As far as I could see, there was no affection between them. If anything, it was contempt he felt for her.

It was his friend Pete who filled me in about that a little later on. Evidently, Dave wanted his freedom to do as he liked. From what I learnt later, that freedom always came at a risk – he was just too conceited to see it. He knew that his mother wouldn't interfere with the sort of things he was getting up to, Pete explained. He also said that Sophia's father owned the building company that had put up all the new houses in the area. That was why Jacqui had been given one. I should think he could hardly wait to get her and Sophia into it. From what I heard, he finally wanted to wash his hands of her and her son.

I wasn't that interested then to ask more questions, I had reached the age where I was coping with a few other small problems that seemed overwhelmingly large to me. I had woken up to stomach pains, gone to the loo and realised from the stain on my pyjamas that my periods had started. Luckily, Mum had explained it all to me a couple of months before she died. I knew all about sanitary towels and how she had said there were always some in their bedroom for when I needed them.

When Dad went out, I had a look for them. I was really worried when I couldn't find any there – he must have got rid of them when he emptied her chest of drawers and cleared out her wardrobe. I felt sad that the only things of hers left were some pieces of jewellery that I had seen her often wear. Her wedding and engagement rings hardly left her hands. Dad had told me more than once that, when I was old enough, I would have them. That day never came, but that's in a later part of my story.

I stood in the bedroom that once two people had slept in and asked myself whether he had forgotten that he had a daughter. Didn't he know that I might need those things that he had got rid of? I mean, he should have known that I wouldn't stay a little girl forever, shouldn't he? At that age I was too embarrassed to ask him where I could get the sanitary pads that Mum had told me about. Now what was I to do?

What do you think, stupid? I told myself. *Go over to Anne's, she'll know what to do.*

'Of course, I'll get some for you,' she said the moment I told her what the problem was. 'I've only got to go to the local chemist to get them. You wait here and I'll be back soon.'

I would say that once your periods begin is a bit of a peculiar time for girls. Right up to then, you feel like you're a child, but then overnight, you're starting to transition into becoming a young woman. That meant I had to be more independent and not expect adults to sort everything out for me. And if I had forgotten those feelings, having a teenage daughter so reminds me of that time.

Not much longer after that visit to Anne, I began to notice other little changes in my body. One of them told me that it was time for me to wear a bra. When I asked Dad if he had noticed that I had lost a little weight, he gave me a brief look and simply said, 'Yes, you have. I'm pleased.' Still, he seemed in a reasonable enough mood so, without mentioning underwear, I just asked him if I could get some new clothes as most of mine, which had been straining at the seams, were now too big.

'Yes, all right,' was all he said.

On the Saturday morning I was relieved as he handed me an envelope with a decent wad of money in it.

'There's enough in there for you to buy some new clothes and you're going with Anne, aren't you?' When I said yes, he made quite a hurtful remark: 'Then you won't be coming back with anything that doesn't suit you.'

So that was another shopping trip with Anne. This time we had coffee out and chatted away cheerfully about what we had to buy.

'You've lost a lot of weight,' she told me.

'Good, I tried to,' I said, though that was only partly true. Giving half of those takeaways to Sophia had meant the pounds started coming off. *Still*, I thought, *best keep quiet about that*. I knew Anne wouldn't be happy with me spending so much time with a woman like Jacqui.

I was really pleased with the way I was looking and, once I tried my new underwear on, I kept one of my new bras on straight away. Anne had got the shop to measure me properly and the assistant explained the importance of buying the right size bra. She also gave me advice on washing them and I was given a leaflet on 'your first bra'. With it on, I definitely felt that I was no longer a child.

Now for a pair of new jeans and some tops, I decided.

When I pulled them on and walked out of the changing room to show Anne, she beamed at me.

'Goodness, you do look like your mother at your age,' she said.

I'm not going to let Donna and her friends treat me like a child now, I told myself as we made our way home. *They might be older than me, but I'm a teenager now too.*

A few days later when we were all at Jacqui's, I refused to have another glass of lemonade. 'I'm old enough now to drink the same as you,' I said as firmly as I could. 'I've got enough money in my purse to chip in as well so you can all stop thinking of me as a silly little girl who has to be given soft drinks.'

They all laughed at this outburst, but it was done in a friendly manner.

'Wondered when you were going to wake up and become one of us,' Donna said merrily.

'Yup, I could tell by the tightness of your shirt that you were growing up,' said one of the boys. 'Here's your drink then,' he added and, still smiling, he poured some cider into a glass and passed it over to me. I didn't know then, and I don't know now, where all the booze came from. It was always stored in big stone jars but I never found out where Jacqui got it from. I do know that it was a lot stronger than the cider that comes in the bottles from the off licence because I can remember feeling dizzy after just a few gulps.

The first couple of times that I was drinking cider, I was sensible enough not to down too many glasses but, naturally, the time came when that sense disappeared. I was still a few weeks short of turning thirteen on the night when I got myself really drunk. There was a kind of party going to take place at Jacqui's, which I had been invited to. I had to find an excuse not to go home that night. Jacqui told me I could sleep there, so in other words, I could doss down on some cushions, then get myself cleaned up and go home on the Saturday morning.

'Your dad wouldn't be happy if you didn't get home after midnight now, would he?'

'No, Jacqui, he wouldn't,' I said.

If he was in and not too pissed himself to notice, I thought, but didn't say it.

'I'll tell him I'm staying over at a friend's house then,' I added.

'Which you will be, so you're not telling a lie.'

When I told Dad that I was staying with a girl who was having a birthday party, he didn't seem bothered at all and even gave me some money in case I changed my mind and wanted to get a taxi home. 'You might want to buy a present for her as well as a card,' he added as he peeled off a few more notes and slipped another £20 into my hand. At least he was generous with money – I nearly always had a few notes in my purse.

The evening before the party, I found the small travelling bag that I had taken with me as hand luggage on my holiday in Turkey. In it went my newest pair of jeans and the pale blue shirt I had also got with Anne. I had a toothbrush and toothpaste and some underwear, and planned to change once school was over.

The moment our last class came to an end, into the loo I went. I could see in the mirror that, once I had wriggled into my jeans and shirt, I liked what I saw because my shape had changed quite a bit. I was curvier, the bra was giving my breasts more definition and my weight was down even more. Most probably because I was eating less and Dad had stopped buying me cakes and biscuits, which he had showered me with after Mum died.

We had to waste a bit of time before we arrive at Jacqui's so Donna and I went to a café, where we met up with some of her friends. 'You're looking good,' she told me as we walked together to the café. That compliment made me puff up a bit. *Right*, I thought, *I'm going to put that lipstick on*, and borrowing a mirror from Donna, I coated my lips with a pale pink. Looking at myself in the mirror, I liked what I saw reflecting back at me.

I can remember that night pretty well, though there are bits of it that I wish I couldn't. Sophia was with a child minder, which was just as well as the house became both crowded and noisy. As well as the usual teenage crowd that followed Donna, Dave and Pete had invited a few friends too and, for once, there was plenty to eat.

'Help yourselves,' Jacqui told everyone as she pointed to the kitchen table, which was laden with dishes of food as well as bottles of wines, spirits and jugs of alcoholic cocktails.

When I say I can remember that night, I mean that I can quite clearly picture the first couple of hours. There was loud music playing, some dancing that we swayed to, lots of chat and some more compliments about how I was looking, which pleased me no end.

The trouble with young drinkers is that one drink too many can stop any sense that is left in their heads from working. I must have downed another one and then goodness knows how many more came after that.

I have a vague recollection of my legs feeling wobbly and my stomach telling me that it was on its way to chucking up everything I had swallowed. At least I managed to get up those stairs and made it to the bathroom. Maybe the downstairs loo was occupied, or perhaps I decided that it was not big enough to throw up in. All I can say is that it was a good thing I didn't fall down those stairs.

My hair was really quite long then and, as I bent down over the loo, I felt someone holding it back for me as I retched and retched and probably groaned as well. When a hand rubbed my back a little, I automatically thought it must be one of my friends. I wiped my mouth with the back of my hand and thanked them before, with a gigantic effort, I managed to straighten up. It was then that I found myself looking into Pete's eyes.

'You'll be all right now,' he told me as he passed me a wet flannel and a big bottle of cold water. 'Thought you might need this: rinse your mouth out a few times and then drink as much as you can. You'll be better sleeping it off now. Go into Sophia's room and I'll look in a few times to make sure you're all right.'

Despite being pretty embarrassed that an older, good-looking boy had helped me, I was grateful too. I could hardly believe he was being so kind to me. That was the beginning of what I believed then was a friendship. I had no idea that he had very different plans for me.

Had I known that and been more worldly-wise, maybe my life would have turned out differently.

15

Reading the next two diary entries written by my younger self brought back so many memories of the months after that girl threw up so much when she first consumed alcohol when she was nearly thirteen to when she turned fourteen.

Funny, isn't it, how boys can ignore us one day and the next use every excuse to come near us? It must be something that happens when they're around thirteen or fourteen that awakens their interest in the opposite sex.

Having lost that podgy, comfort-eating weight and grown my thick dark hair long, I found that suddenly, they wanted to be friendly. To be honest, I liked it! I mean, what teenage girl who has been ignored for over a year wouldn't? Not that any of the ones who sauntered over in my direction impressed me much.

The boy I keep hearing the other girls talking about is not one of those young ones with spots on their chins and voices that are breaking, but Pete, who is in the sixth form. I also hear rumours that he's a bad boy and yet they fancy him rotten. Talk about flirting with him, they are all pouty lips and big eyes meeting his at every opportunity they can. If he had asked any one of them out, as he did me, I think they might have wet themselves with excitement. I almost can't believe it that the boy who all the other girls think of as hot, asked *me* out the Monday after that party. And he had seen me drunk and embarrassing myself. Seems he didn't care about my disgusting retching when he strolled up to me in the school yard.

'Hi Amy,' he says, 'how about we go out for a coffee after school instead of going to Jacqui's? I know quite a nice café not far from here.'

As I look down at that dog-eared black exercise book that lays in my lap, I remember that day in minute detail. How I stood smiling up at him and shyly agreed. Unlike the other girls my age, I thought he was a bit too old for me. I didn't think he was 'my type', whatever that was. I liked boys with tousled hair who never bothered about looking smart. That didn't stop me saying yes though. Out of school, Pete wore sporty tracksuits with designer brand labels, which I thought were the epitome of style. As for messy hair? Not that boy: he must have gone to the barber regularly. His black hair was cut in what my dad always referred to as a short back and sides. Not once in the time that I knew him did it appear to need a trim.

So if he's not your type, why are you meeting up with him? Was it because you believed he would make a good friend? The answer is that I want to make the girls who had been horrid to me jealous! I could get what they dreamed of having!

That made me smile when I read it, as did the next piece:

Out of the corner of my eye I could see a small group of girls looking over at me while Pete was standing next to me, talking. The moment he walked away, one of them, who I really disliked as she had more than once mocked my weight gain, walked over. There she is by my side, trying to look as friendly as possible. I try to look the same so that she can think I'm pleased to see her. Well, of course I was, but not for the reasons she might think.

She chatters a little about nothing I find interesting until she gets to the real reason of why she's come over to me as if I didn't know – 'What was that all about with Pete? He looked quite serious.'

Great, I think, *now I can really wind her up!*

'Oh, it was just him inviting me to go out with him after school,' I say as nonchalantly as I can while gleefully tossing that long mane of mine. Oh, diary, you should have seen her face drop before she walked back to her friends. There they are, heads together as she tells them what she's just heard. Heads keep rising from the huddle and look my way! When all the classes are finished, there they are again standing by the exit gate, watching as Pete and I walk out together. I hope they feel sick with jealousy that it's me and not one of them by his side.

Of course I can remember what would be called my first date. The café Pete took me to was a pretty one, it did great cakes and it took all my willpower to say no.

'No more sugary stuff for me,' I told him.

'Amy, you look great,' he said with a really warm smile as I felt his hand go over mine. 'I like you in those jeans of yours, they really suit you.'

That was one of the rare times when I hadn't brought a change of clothes because I was going straight home after school. I had too much homework to stay out late. We were both in our uniforms as we chatted in the café, even though I felt more like a grown-up when I was not wearing school uniform and I must say he also looked more interesting when he was wearing his own out-of-school clothes.

That afternoon I was surprised by how much I enjoyed his company. What I know now is that he was determined to make me fall for him. Still, not knowing anything about dating and the manipulation that can come with it, I found myself having a good time. He was really good fun and I felt we had lots in common. I know now that he did his best to make me feel that way. We talked about Jacqui's house, music we liked, even books we had read, but nothing about our respective home lives. He was smart enough not to bring that up. When he looked at his watch and saw that I didn't have long to catch my bus home, he asked if I would like to go out one evening to a restaurant. That sounded good to me, so I must have smiled away and said yes.

He then gave me a little advice about being able to pass for eighteen. 'It's a nice restaurant,' he told me, 'so there's no fuss about you being there, but if you want to have a glass of wine, then you need to look a little older. I suggest you wear what you wore at Jacqui's and put on a little more make-up. Then they'll believe you're old enough to have a drink.'

My feeling now is that he didn't want people wondering what someone of his age was doing out with an obviously underage girl but back then I believed it was only about me having a glass of wine with my meal, which, of course, made me feel rather sophisticated.

So I did as he had suggested and went shopping for make-up, getting mascara, eye liner and a darker colour lipstick. Luckily, like most young girls, I had watched Mum putting on make-up. She only wore it on special occasions and tried to make it look as natural as possible. 'A little of everything is the best,' she had told me. I practised doing my make-up different ways until I thought I had got it just right. I told Dad that I was going out with a friend's family for her birthday when I explained that I would be out that night. He just nodded and offered me money for a taxi home.

Pete made appreciative noises when he saw me, which made me blush with pleasure. He knew what sort of food I liked, probably by seeing the takeaways I gave to Sophia, and had booked a table in a really upmarket Thai restaurant. In his jeans and leather jacket, he looked really gorgeous – and

I could tell our waitress thought that too because she was all over him. I felt like the luckiest girl in the world.

To my relief, no one looked suspicious about my age. Yes, of course we had a great evening and yes, I had that glass of wine or even two. And as to be expected by the end of the night, I was totally smitten. He ordered me a taxi home at a sensible hour. Did we kiss? Yes, we did but, as the taxi was waiting, it was quite quick, although it still made me tingle all over. As the taxi drove me home, I knew that I was grinning from ear to ear.

That was the beginning of us seeing each other regularly. It was also the beginning of everyone being friendly to me. Any jealousy from the other girls was well hidden. It was being with Pete that had changed my life, or so I believed then and I was convinced that it was all for the better. He was the first boy I had ever dated, and what does a young teenage girl who is spending time with a boy several years older than herself do? She tries to act like a grown-up.

It must have been a few weeks after I had first gone out with him that Pete invited me to spend a Saturday evening at his house: 'Mum and Dad are away for the weekend so we can chill out. I've got some great music that you'll love hearing, plus I've some decent wine upstairs in my room. Unless you have other plans, that is?' I could hardly say I had nothing else to do except tidy my bedroom and the kitchen, could I? Instead, I just stammered, 'That sounds great.'

It was a little later when a small niggling worry surfaced. We had kissed a lot during the times I spent with him, but kissing in the park or on street corners was one thing, whereas kissing in a room where there would only be the two of us was very different. Did I really want it to go further than that? *Don't be silly*, my devious inner voice told me, *he won't make you do anything you don't want to do*. Well, that inner voice of mine certainly got that wrong, though he was far too careful to do what he had planned that first time.

All Dad knew about my going out that Saturday was that I was meeting up with some friends. He told me to have a good time without asking any questions. So I took a bus, still feeling a little apprehensive in one way and excited in another. I spent the time looking out of the window and, when the bus reached my destination, Pete was waiting for me at the bus stop. He gave me a hug and told me I was looking good then led the way to his house, saying it wasn't too far.

I was impressed by my first sight of his home when we reached it: an imposing three-storey house, lying a little back from the road.

'I've got the whole of the attic; it's almost like having my own flat.' The hall, I noticed, had an amazing number of pictures hanging in it and the wide staircase was covered in thick deep pink carpet.

'Up we go,' he told me.

My eyes opened wide when I walked in. It was the smartest bedroom I had ever seen. The windows at the back of his room overlooked a beautiful and colourful garden and were huge, letting in lots of light. The room was painted white, which gave a clear background for all the posters of different bands he had on the walls. The flooring was a light-coloured wood with several sheepskin rugs laid down on it. Like Jacqui's big room, there was a pile of floor cushions that could be sat on, next to those windows. In the centre was a large bed, larger than Mum and Dad's at home, and opposite it was a television, which was hung on the wall. There was only one chair that had piles of stuff on it and in front of it was a small table covered in magazines that were all about cars. That was the messy part of the room, the rest of it was tidy.

My eyes followed him as he turned on the music and I heard pleasant moody sounds coming from a very expensive Bose system. 'Like that?' he asked and I answered, 'I really do. It's the kind of music that I love listening to.' He then went over to his tiny fridge and took out a bottle of white wine. After pouring two glasses, he brought them over to where I was standing: 'Hold them, will you?' he said as he put them both in my hands and then he chucked everything on the chair onto the floor. 'Now that's better. Sit down, Amy,' he added as he grabbed his drink and sat down in the only chair.

I suppose I'll have to sit on the bed then, I thought as I perched myself on it.

He lifted his glass up into the air, 'Cheers, beautiful,' and the words made me giggle a little. It didn't take long for my glass to be nearly empty and, seeing it, he went back to the fridge and filled it right to the top. By then the combination of wine and having the music in the background made me feel both relaxed and happy.

'Like to smoke a little?' he asked as he opened a tin of tobacco and began mixing it with small flakes that he shaved from a small brown lump of what I already knew to be dope. 'No harm in taking it,' Jacqui had told me more than once when I smelt the distinctive perfumed fumes coming from the settee where she was lying. 'It makes people feel peaceful.'

As I had never put a cigarette near my mouth, I was very unsure, mainly because smoking cigarettes was something Mum hated so much: 'They're bad for you and I loathe the stink of them,' she had told me more than once. Even though she was no longer around, I did try to stick to the advice she had given me. That evening, though, I didn't have the guts to say no. I wanted Pete to see me as a grown-up who had been smoking cigarettes and joints for ages. I was convinced that he would just see me as a baby and think less of me if I said no. So instead of doing what my inner voice told me to do, I nodded and said yes as nonchalantly as I could.

As I choked on my first puff, I couldn't stop coughing. Pete patted my back, poured me some more wine and said, 'Don't inhale so fast. Just a tiny puff and suck it deep into your lungs.'

'OK,' I managed to say as I worked at getting my breath back.

After he had taken a long drag, it was passed back to me. This time I tried to do as he had done and at least I didn't choke.

The sound of the music seemed to become even dreamier after I finally managed to inhale a reasonable amount. I felt so comfortable when he moved over to the bed and put his arms around me and held me close.

'You're so beautiful,' he told me as one of his fingers went under my chin, raising my face up a little higher. I gazed back into those green eyes of his.

'You're the good-looking one,' I said. 'All the girls at school say that about you.'

'They might, but you're the only one I want to be with,' he told me just a second before he pulled me closer and his lips met mine. Swinging his legs onto the bed, he pulled me up beside him and told me again that he thought I was beautiful. I nestled up to him and, when both his arms wrapped around me, he kissed me again.

'Those other girls will be so jealous if I tell them what we've been doing,' I giggled as I looked up at him.

'Maybe you'd better not tell anyone then,' he told me. 'Best if we just keep this to ourselves. Don't want you getting un-popular again, now do we?'

'No, I suppose I'd better keep quiet then.'

'Good girl,' he said before giving me another long kiss.

Oh yes, I remember that evening very well. He didn't make any more moves. To me, it seemed that he did all the right things. He told me that I'd better not be too late going home and that I should tidy myself up a little and he would walk me to the bus stop.

'Don't want your father getting angry if you're late, now do we?'

'No, I don't,' I answered without saying what I was really thinking, *that's if my dad's in, that is.*

I can picture myself wreathed in smiles of happiness after being kissed by my first boyfriend. As I got ready to leave, I was even happier when he said that his parents were away the next weekend too: 'You can stay here if you can think of a good excuse to give your dad. There are lots of things we can do round here. Go for walks, eat out and listen to music.'

Spending a whole weekend alone with him sounded absolutely wonderful to me.

'Oh, I'm sure Dad won't mind. I'll just say I'm spending it with one of my friends.'

Another cuddle came my way before he took my hand and walked me down to the bus stop. He waited with me until the bus came. We talked and kissed all the while and, as the bus pulled away, he waved goodbye once I was seated. For the whole of that short journey, I was floating on a rosy cloud fuelled by something I thought of as love, although in reality it was white wine and my first experience of cannabis.

I had no idea that the next time I would be with him would also herald the first of too many of my encounters with the police.

16

The following Friday, when I was supposed to be meeting Pete after classes finished, I received a note from Jacqui during one of our breaks. She must have paid a taxi firm to bring it over and give it to one of the seniors to give to me. It was quite a stern-faced male prefect who, looking rather curious, handed it to me: 'I was told by a driver to give this to you when you were on your break,' he announced stiffly before walking away.

Thinking it might have come from Pete because I hadn't seen him at school all day, I just about ripped it open. I felt a wave of disappointment when I saw the signature at the bottom of the page was Jacqui's and not his – I was supposed to be meeting up with him later. *Anyhow, let's see what Jacqui has to say*, I thought. I was somewhat puzzled when I saw that she was asking me to come over to hers when I finished school. That was unusual because she never seemed to mind when it was any of us turned up. I wondered if something had happened or if she or Sophia was ill, so I decided I had better go and, anyhow, she might know where Pete was. *Maybe he's over there already*, I thought.

The questions circled around in my head because I was concerned about Pete's whereabouts and at the time this was far more important to me than finding out the reason why Jacqui wanted to see me. Nothing like being keen on a boy to make us rather selfish, is there? That's teenagers for you, especially an infatuated one.

The moment our last lesson ended, I grabbed my satchel and my rucksack with clothes, make-up and toiletries in it and rushed to the toilets so I could change. A few minutes later, I was on my way, full of anticipation.

I was pretty startled when I got near Jacqui's house and found that, for the first time since I had known her, she was not lying on the couch with a drink in her hand. Instead, she must have been watching through the window so that she could see me coming. She opened the door when I was only a couple of feet away, which made me realise that she was really eager to see me. That worried me a little. It was so out of character that I was pretty certain that something was wrong – I just hoped it was nothing to do with Sophia.

'Oh, Amy, I'm so pleased you've come. Come in,' she said and I could see that she had been crying, which was not like her at all.

I didn't need to ask what the problem was. As soon as she put a glass of cider in my hand and topped her own glass up, she began to tell me everything that had happened that day. I felt a bit better when I found out that it had nothing to do with Sophia because I interrupted her to ask where she was.

'I thought it better if she stayed with her child minder today, there's just too much going on here today,' she explained.

I couldn't help thinking why she was so anxious to see me and what was happening? It took just a few seconds for me to establish that it was all to do with her son: 'Dave's on his way to prison now. He was arrested, taken to court and I thought he'd get off. It's not as though it's a serious crime, is it?'

'No,' I said, even though I didn't have an inkling of what exactly Dave had been caught doing. She then gave enough detail for my heart to sink. Did it mean that Pete had been involved as well? Wasn't he Dave's closest friend and didn't they get up to mischief together? It wasn't something that I had ever asked Pete about, but there were enough rumours around the school that had told me there might be a risk of him also being involved. The thought of Pete being arrested as well put fear in me.

Jacqui, seeing my expression, gave me a little smile. 'Oh, don't look so worried, love! Pete was lucky, he wasn't caught and Dave didn't shop him. Luckily for Pete, my Dave's a loyal friend, isn't it?'

'What happened?'

'They stole another car. I think the police must have been watching them for a while.'

'Why?'

'Why do you think? It's not just the odd car they steal, and it's not all they get up to either.'

For Jacqui to tell me all that so calmly really shocked me. I had thought all along that she had no idea what her son was up to. Not that I had been aware of them stealing cars.

The rumours at school were just that they got up to a few illegal things. I had naively thought that they were just selling weed, maybe pills too. No wonder I was wide-eyed with shock at what she was telling me.

'So, where's Dave now?'

'He was in court this morning and was sentenced. Pete was there too, but not in the dock. He was only listening so he could hone me when the trial was over and let me know the result, though I was pretty sure that this time he wouldn't be coming home. Even his barrister wasn't hopeful.'

It was on the tip of my tongue to ask why she hadn't gone but she swiftly explained: 'I should have gone – I always did before, but I wanted Pete's conscience to tell him that it was partly his fault. If he has one, that is. I hoped that sitting in a court where his best friend was being cross-examined in front of a magistrate and whoever is in there gawking because they want some entertainment would make him feel guilty.'

She got up then and topped up both our glasses.

'He's only been sentenced for a few months,' she told me once she sat down again. 'Even so, it means he'll have a criminal record, which he can't get rid of. Before it was the juvenile court and he got a caution, not even a suspended sentence. Now this will make it more difficult for him to get a job in the future.

'I'm sure the police were furious that the sentence was so short and even more so when they weren't able to charge Pete as well. They took him in – not the first time, let me add – questioned him with his fancy solicitor there and got nowhere. They must have done their best to get Dave to tell them that there were two of them, not just one stealing the car but my son kept his mouth shut so there was nothing they could do. I expect they were beside themselves when they were told that the only fingerprints found were my son's.

'Now I want you to understand something, Amy. They will keep watching Pete and anyone who appears to be close to him,' she said with a warning stare. 'Do you get that?'

And I did, up to a point, but my mind was focused on wanting to know where Pete was now and it seemed as though Jacqui was more intent on having another drink than saying much more. My glass was topped up again, as was hers. I sipped my drink while I tried to pluck up enough courage to ask where Pete was. Just as I was seconds off from opening my mouth, the phone rang. I watch as she grabbed it and heard her saying that Dave should be much more careful in the future before adding, 'And so should you be, otherwise you'll end up in the same place as him. Not a good idea to start your adult life inside, is it? It certainly won't be for my son and, let's face it, you might have been going down with him had he spoken up about you.'

Those last sentences told me that it was Pete she was talking to. I was on my third drink by then and dying to get hold of that phone, but I could hardly interrupt. I just hoped she would pass the phone over to me once she had finished listening to whatever he was saying.

Just as I was getting impatient, I heard her voice rising: 'Yeah, she's here. What do you want her for?'

Whatever he was saying on the phone was not making her smile. If anything, I could see that she was rather annoyed.

'That was Pete – I expect you guessed that. He's coming over a little later. That'll please you, won't it? But do you remember what I said, Amy?'

'That the police might be watching anyone he's close to,' I repeated.

'That's right, so you need to watch out. Look, I've only told you this because I care about you and I want you to be careful.'

Now, with the benefit of hindsight, I can understand what Jacqui was trying to do. She did not trust Pete, and she clearly saw me as still very young and under his influence. That was the reason she had asked me to visit – she could see trouble coming my way if I didn't take heed of her warning. Now, all I can say was that she was right – spot-on, in fact. If only I hadn't been so infatuated.

Like most people who visited her house, my impression was that she was well-liked but not respected. I must admit that I felt the same. The problem with Jacqui was that she was seen as the town's alcoholic, which made her the wrong person for someone like me to listen to. Especially as, over the time that I had visited her, I had seen that she was not fussy about who came along and what the crowd of youngsters got up to.

Instead, I just nodded, had another drink and all that advice flew out of my head the instant Pete walked in with a carrier bag full of bottles of cider. The moment I saw him, I felt a smile stretching my mouth.

'Hello there, beautiful,' he said casually as though nothing had gone wrong that day.

Silly me, I actually felt excited at what I thought was him being daring.

'I'm sorry Dave got caught, I really am,' he told Jacqui as he dumped the cider in front of her.

More drinks were poured. Jacqui was already pretty pissed and my head was spinning. I thought Pete's must be as well as his eyes were unusually bright. Though come to think of it, I had only seen him knocking back one glass.

Pulling a chair over next to mine, he took hold of my hand.

'It's been a tough day,' he said.

Had I been sensible, I would have decided right then that I didn't want to mix with crooks but no, I was too impressed that, bad boy or not, all the girls seemed to fancy him, but it was me he had chosen. After another round of drinks, he said, 'Come on, let's go back to my house now.'

Once we were outside, he walked over to a car and opened the door.

'Come on, get in,' he said.

'Is this one you've stolen?'

'Of course.'

17

The next diary covered a time that I was dreading having to revisit. There are pages in it where I write about my love for Pete, whereas my adult self really despises him. He's someone I have tried to block from my thoughts for many years. I'm tempted to rip these pages full of my schoolgirl naivety out, but instead, I flick through them until I come to the part of the diary which tells of my first encounter with the police. Here, I write about my feelings and what I went through.

I'm not really thinking much, my legs are a bit wobbly and as for my thoughts, they're pretty wonky as well. Pete gives me a gentle push to get me in the car while I'm still asking myself whether this is a joke or not. He wouldn't steal a car just outside of Jacqui's, would he? I ask him again and he laughs. 'It's not mine, I haven't got a car yet,' he says as he turns on the engine and puts his foot down on the accelerator. When I realise it's not a joke, I'm scared. Part of me wants to scream at him to stop and let me out and the other part thinks it's all a bit of an adventure.

It didn't take long for me to wish I had done just that. Hadn't lots of the girls at school told me he was a bad boy, even though they all fancied him? I can't help it, I'm so proud it's me he likes the most and I don't want him to think I'm a cowardly little girl.

If I was slightly scared, then I'm much more frightened when we reach the end of the estate and I see a cop car pulling up in front of us, blue lights flashing. Pete had to slam on the brakes fast to avoid running into the back of it. He swore and turned off the engine.

The car doors open and two big, beefy men in uniform walk towards us. I feel sick with nerves when I see the scowls on their faces.

'You two get out,' was all they said when Pete opened his window to see what they wanted. He began to say something about the car, which sounded as though he had every right to be in it. The policeman just told him to shut up and get out. The bigger one of the two opened the passenger door, leaned down and grabbed my arm, pulling me out. 'You stink of booze,' he tells me. 'So why aren't I surprised? A little drunken thief, aren't you?'

I try to say I'm not, but his grip is so tight it's hurting me. He tells me he knows my type and he's taking me in too. His huge hands are still clasping my arm as he drags me over to the police car and throws me in the back seat. The other cop pulls Pete's arms behind his back and once handcuffed, he pushes him in beside me.

'Nice and cosy for you two,' he smirks. My face must be burning and I can see people in the road staring at us. I hear Pete telling the cop to leave me alone.

Another 'shut up' comes out of the fatter one's mouth.

All I'm thinking then is why didn't they just ask us to get in the car? They only had to tell us to do that and we would have done so. There's no reason, except they seem to like using their muscles to scare and intimidate us.

Over my teenage years I was to learn that there they are certain types of men who enjoy humiliating vulnerable people: it makes them feel powerful. Those two policemen must have known roughly how young I was then, even though they pretended not to. They clearly just wanted to take revenge on Pete because they were not able to get him into court and sentenced for the theft of the car with Dave, which although they had no proof, they were convinced that he was involved in.

I can remember how frightened I was and my whole body must have been shaking with fear. Pete kept whispering that everything would be all right, but I was in such a state of shock, I couldn't take a word in. I didn't know that they had to treat a minor differently to an adult as I only had a limited of knowledge about the law, mostly gained from TV shows and many of those were American. In my head, as we were driven to the police station, I believed that we were going to be locked up and sent to prison.

Pete tries again to get through to me as he whispers in
my ear that the car was not a stolen one, it was Dave's
and he had permission to use it.

I should think the police already knew that. It was not the
theft of the car that must have interested them, but a totally
different crime they believed they could prove. They had only
used the fact that Pete didn't have the documentation for the
car as an excuse to bring him in. Of course, they were totally
out of order as now I know you have a fixed time to present
them at the police station.

They clearly also knew that I was underage and they must
have seen me with Pete more than once. I never did find out
who the spy was, probably someone who had it in for Pete.
I didn't realise it then but now I know that, if I was Pete's
girlfriend, which they believed, then all they had to do was
to get me to admit we had had sex and then they could
charge him with having sex with a minor. Their plan was to
ask a friendly-looking policewoman to take care of me. The
contrast between how they had treated me and how nice and
friendly she was would cause many a frightened underage
girl to trust her – and trust would make her answer questions
more truthfully.

I can still picture in my head how that plan was put into
action. Did it work? Not really, though it might have been
better for me if it had. Maybe then that would have been the
first and last time I encountered those two policemen.

Meeting those two policemen that day was the beginning of my path of bad luck. It was as if they had a photo of me behind their eyes. Each time they saw me somewhere in town, they managed to find different ways of harassing me.

Anyway, I'd better go back to the part in the diary when my younger self not only wrote about Pete and I being frog-marched into the police station, but what happened there.

Luckily, being so frightened had sobered me up enough to stop me being careless with the answers to the questions that came my way. It was Pete the police wanted to deal with first, or rather, they wanted to separate us as fast as they could. I could hear him saying that he was allowed one call and that would be to his family's solicitor. The answer to that was the police would arrange that a little later once he had been questioned. All their phone lines were busy, they explained: 'Seems it's a day for crooks to be out.'

Pete looked worried then. He didn't want to spend the rest of the day in a cell, but that's what happened.

Glancing again at the diary causes more memories of that day to return. I remember Pete saying, 'Why don't you let Amy go? She's done nothing wrong. I was only giving her a lift home.' That was the last sentence I heard him say. Mocking glances were exchanged and one of the policemen grabbed hold of his arm and escorted him away to an interview room.

'You wait here,' the second officer told me as he indicated a seat in the charge office before he went through a door with NO UNAUTHORISED PERSONNEL on it. Not that I could have made a run for it, there were another couple of police-men there giving me curious sideways glances.

It was such a shame that, back then, I was completely un-aware that I could have walked out.

It was just a few minutes before that door opened again and the policeman came over to me with a young female colleague by his side.

'This is Constable Davies. She's going to interview you,' he told me. 'We only need a few details so mind you tell her the truth, no lies. Understand?'

I could hardly say anything but yes.

I can picture that policewoman now. She gave me a gentle smile and said, 'Just come along with me, Amy. And stop looking so scared. We're just going to have a little talk and there are a few questions I need you to answer, that's all.'

She took me into a small room. Containing only four upright wooden chairs and a table with a small machine on top, it looked cold and bare.

'Are you thirsty?' she asked.

And I was. Fear and too much cider had removed all the moisture from my mouth, making my voice sound scratchy.

'Yes,' I admitted, 'I could do with some water.'

She pressed some sort of button near her and a colleague, who looked even younger than her, appeared pretty quickly.

'Can you get us both some tea and a jug of water, Yvonne,' she asked. 'Best bring some biscuits as well – Amy here looks as though she could do with something a little sweet.'

'Will do,' she replied and, after shooting a friendly smile in my direction, she disappeared but it didn't take long for her to reappear, carrying a tray with everything Constable Davies had requested.

I wonder why they're being so nice to me, I thought. But hadn't I learned enough to know that being nice can be an act purely to make us trust someone, such as a teacher who wants to find out why our homework wasn't done? Remembering that put me on my guard. After all, that policeman, being a sergeant and more senior to her, must have given her a few instructions before I was handed over. That was enough to make me keep my head down and look as mild as possible.

Constable Davies asked what age I was, noting that I looked pretty young to her.

'I'll be thirteen in a couple of weeks,' I told her and I saw an expression flashing in her eyes that told me she was pleased with my answer. I watched her write that down before asking me for my address.

Better not give her mine, I immediately thought and so I gave her Jacqui's instead. I certainly did not want the police getting in touch with Dad. Probably not the best move, considering Jacqui must have been known to the police, but I was desperate.

Of course, that policewoman should have told me that she needed to do just that. The law states that a suitable adult must be with an underage child who is being interviewed. As those two policemen had no intention of getting me a chaperone, I suppose she was being careful with the questions she had been told to ask me.

If anyone, such as a parent or even worse, a solicitor, had tackled that policewoman about being in a room with me without a suitable adult, she could just say that we had only been chatting and the tape recorder was not switched on. There had been no mention of car theft from any of them – I suppose those questions were being asked of Pete.

Seeing I was upset was the reason she had brought me into the room and got me something to eat and drink so that I stopped being frightened would probably be her explanation.

'How long are we going to be here?' I asked. 'I think neither of us have done anything wrong – that car belonged to his friend.'

'I wouldn't know what it is my colleagues want to ask him,' she told me and I believed her. Now, of course, I know full well that she had been told exactly what they were doing.

The next few questions she put to me would have made it clear, if only I had been a little more knowledgeable.

'They were horrible to us,' I told her and she gave me a sympathetic look.

'I can tell you're close to Pete,' she said. 'How long have you been going out with him?'

That question woke my suspicions a little. Just what was she getting at?

'He's just a friend,' I told her quickly. Maybe *too* quickly for her to believe me.

'He's your boyfriend, isn't he?' she persisted. 'My colleague told me he'd noticed that Pete really cares for you. I'm sure he's very good to you. He's handsome as well, I hear. Don't you feel lucky to have him?'

It was a good thing that, having learnt a lot at Jacqui's, I was smart enough not to say yes to these questions.

'I'm lucky to have him as a friend, but that's all he is,' I told her. 'He was at the same school as me and I got to know him a little more when we were both visiting Mrs Turner.'

'Doesn't Pete take you out sometimes?›

'Not really. He treated me to a meal once and then got me a taxi home, that's all.'

'You haven't slept with him then?' The question just about shot out, making me gasp a little.

'No, of course not. I just told you he was at the same school as me and he's a friend of Mrs Turner.'

'You mean a friend of her son Dave, who has just gone to prison for car theft?'

That stopped me.

'Still, that's not your problem, is it?'

'No, it's not,' I answered with a sigh.

'I have one more thing to ask you: are you still a virgin?'

'Yes, I am,' I said indignantly, for it was still the truth then.

I could tell from the faint smile that came in my direction that she believed me.

'I'm pleased to hear it, Amy. Just stay here, will you? I'll be back in a minute.'

She left the room for a while, doubtless passing on the information she had gleaned to the two officers who had brought me in.

What's going to happen now? I wondered. *Will they tell Dad?*

Just have to wait and see, my inner voice said.

When Constable Davies came back into the room, my heart sank: she was not alone. The policeman who had pulled me out of the car came strutting in behind her with such a look of rage on his face that I knew straight away he was determined to make the rest of that day even worse for me. Constable Davies must have known this as well from the look of concern on her face.

Many years later I found out that the young constable had been new to the force when I first met her. She hadn't thought for one moment that, in the first few months after her training, she would be under the thumbs of two misogynists. Those two bullies had almost scared her enough to make her think of leaving the job. Going against their demands could end the career she had worked so hard to build. She knew from her time at the police training school what the laws of interviewing were, whereas they had almost certainly been ignoring them for so long that they saw breaking the rules as necessary to getting convictions.

The sergeant evidently felt he had made her nervous enough for him to break the law in front of her when he verbally abused me.

'Now, you little liar, it would be better for you if, for once, you told the truth. I know Pete's your boyfriend and what the two of you get up to the moment you're alone together.'

For a moment I froze. Had he seen us kissing somewhere?

Just deny it, my inner voice piped up.

'He's not,' I insisted as firmly as I could muster. 'He's just a friend.'

'Oh, really? So, a good-looking a young man of eighteen decides to be pally with a girl who's not had her thirteenth birthday yet? Come on, Amy, why would that be then? I can only think of one answer: he likes shagging stupid little girls.'

Tell them why you have older friends, my inner voice said. *Mum wouldn't mind, especially if it just helps shut him up.*

'Well, yes, he's been nice to me,' I told them both as innocently as I could. 'He's not the only older person who has been, either. There's a whole group of them who've looked out for me ever since Mum died.'

From the way his face dropped, I could tell that the he knew nothing about my circumstances. Constable Davies looked even more concerned and embarrassed as well.

'When did she die?' she asked, gently stepping in.

'Two years ago, on Mother's Day. I still miss her every day,' I said.

Just the admission brought tears to my eyes with no warning. Even the sergeant looked distinctly uneasy.

Pull your shoulders back and look him in the eye, my inner voice told me. That wasn't easy, but I managed.

'If she was still with us, she would be standing here demanding that I was let go,' I added and, as these words were spoken, I could tell immediately they angered the sergeant.

'That's what you think, Missy. No one else seems bothered about you. Your dad's not been ringing the station to tell us you're not home from school. That's what a worried parent does. Or maybe he's not expecting you and you've been making excuses to stay out late?'

'He doesn't always come home when he's finished work. He has friends he goes out with. He still finds being in the house depressing without Mum in it – I expect he's not got home yet.'

'Like father, like daughter,' he sneered. 'He's out getting pissed as well, is he?'

There was nothing I could say to that and so I looked down, which seemed to make him even more angry. He began almost shouting at me, saying he knew I was sleeping with Pete and I'd better admit it.

'I'm not,' I insisted.

'Oh, yes, I forgot. You're a virgin, aren't you? You told our constable that and now you're telling me the same thing. She might believe you, but I don't. So, what will you say if a doctor comes here and has a nice deep look at your fanny? He'll find out then, won't he?'

It was this last taunt that finally reduced me – tears were rolling down my cheeks. Hearing those words and seeing how her colleague had finally affected me was enough to make Constable Davies move to stand in front of him.

'Stop,' she said quietly before pushing herself up onto her toes and saying something in his ear that I couldn't hear.

He glared at her and then shrugged.

'Get this little brat into a cell and stop pandering to her, will you, Constable? She can stay there until an adult comes and claims her if that's what you want so badly.'

I saw the blush rise on the constable's face. She said nothing more to him, just touched my arm and said, 'Let's go where you can rest a little.'

As we walked to where the cells were located, she explained that the ones for those who were underage were a little different from the others.

'There's not a loo inside these ones. We understand that young people might be too embarrassed to use the one in their cell so all you have to do is press the buzzer and I'll come down to you.'

When we got to the cells, I thought I'd never seen such miserable little places.

'Where's Pete?' I wanted to know.

'He's in an adult cell, which is further up. Look, don't get too stressed, you're not going to be here for long. Pete has rung his solicitor and he'll be acting for you as well so just try and be patient.' Pausing outside a toilet, she added, 'Best go to the loo before we put you in your cell – I've a lot to write up before I can get back for a while.'

No doubt she would have to listen to what the sergeant had to say when she wrote her report. I know now that he wouldn't have wanted her to spend time with me, obviously thinking she was a soft touch.

I had that final pee, which after all the cider was most welcome, while she waited outside the door and then we walked the last few steps into the cell. That moment is certainly one of my sharpest and clearest memories of our arrest.

I was hoping that I wouldn't be there too long but somehow I didn't believe those words of reassurance that Constable Davies had given me: the police wanted me to be miserable Hearing the keys jangle as she walked away was enough to frighten me. I leant against the bars of the cell with my fingers clenching them until I heard a faint click of the door we had come through closing behind her. The only person who seemed to be on my side had gone. All around me was silence, which made me feel so alone, and I hated the fact that I was locked in. Inside the cell was a small window of thick glass high up and a wooden bench with the thinnest, plastic-covered mattress I had ever seen – it was hardly a place I was going to get comfortable in. Instead, I found myself pacing up and down, even though I was feeling exhausted by then.

Telling them about Mum's death had brought back the grief of losing her. I was missing her so much, tears were rolling down my cheeks.

'If only you were still here, Mum, none of this would be happening,' I kept saying as if she could hear me.

Stop crying, my inner voice told me, but this time I really couldn't. All my bravery had disappeared and my legs wobbled as I moved over to the mattress and sank onto it. My hands clasped the horrible green blanket that must have covered so many others and I drew it over my head in despair, not wanting the policemen to hear me crying.

Reading about my younger self in that cell brings back more memories that even now make me feel tearful.

It seemed a long time before I finally heard the jangle of keys and footsteps coming in my direction.

'It's me, Amy,' Constable Davis called out as she got nearer. She unlocked the door, stepped in and to my relief said that I was free to go now and so was Pete: he and his solicitor were waiting for me.

When I stood up and she saw how much I must have been crying, she placed an arm around my shoulder.

'Come on, no more crying. Let's go to that loo again so you can give your face a wash, then I'll take you up to them.'

So I splashed as much cold water on my face as I could, ran my fingers through my hair and then followed her up to where the solicitor and Pete were.

'Make sure you don't come back in here, Amy,' the constable whispered in my ear.

'I will,' I promised and somehow managed to hold my head up high.

18

Pete smiled at me as best as he could when Constable Davies and I reached him and his solicitor. I saw a flash of anger on the solicitor's face as, when he was introduced to me, he could tell by those puffy eyes of mine that I had been crying.

'Are you all right, Amy?' he asked. By the look of concern on both the constable's face and his, neither of them seemed to think I was.

'I'm all right now,' I answered, wishing Pete would put his arms round me and hug me hard. He didn't, of course; he just patted me on the shoulder saying he hoped I was getting over my horrible experience in the police cell.

'I'm trying to,' was all I said.

'Let's get you both out of here. Constable, can you return any of my clients' possessions that you are holding?' Jeremy spoke with such authority that this was done swiftly and within minutes we were free to go.

'Thank goodness for fresh air,' sighed Pete as we walked out.

'Now, Amy,' Jeremy said to me, 'how tired are you? Are you too tired to eat?'

'No,' I replied, smiling up at him.

'Good, I know I don't even have to ask Pete. There's a place I know where we can relax a little and you two can eat as much as you want. I'm sure you must be thirsty as well as hungry,' he added.

In a way, all I wanted was to have a shower and wash the smell of that blanket off me, crawl into bed and sleep and try to push everything that had happened that evening behind me. I was past being hungry, although the solicitor was right about me being thirsty. Pete was looking completely unperturbed by the ordeal and wide awake, perhaps also very happy at the thought of having a decent meal.

'All sounds great, Jeremy,' he said cheerfully. Considering that he, too, had been locked up for hours, there was no sign of any stress on him, I noticed, while I still felt very shaky and emotional.

'We'll take my car. I can see that Amy looks a little tired so I don't think walking there is a good idea.' He turned to me then, adding in a very kind and reassuring way, 'Some food and a little conversation will start to make you feel better.'

It was these remarks then and on those times when I met him later that told me Pete's solicitor had a compassionate side. I could also tell that he wanted to do his utmost for his clients and that was the side of him I came to like. The other side of him – the business one that was meticulous in the questions he wanted answers to – was the one I learned to respect.

That evening, he was as tactful as he could be in the way he put the questions he asked me.

There was something about his personality that made me feel comfortable. Not that I thought then that this was not going to be the only time I would meet him. I can't remember now just how many times I did meet him, but far too many, I can assure you.

The place he took us to was clearly one he used often both for meetings with clients and more social meals as I could tell straight away that all the waiters knew him. When I heard the waiter say, 'Your usual table, sir?' I guessed that he must have requested, more than once, to have the quietest spot in the restaurant. We were taken to a table as far away as possible from the other more packed ones where people sat chatting away over dinner. He must have booked it before we were released because it was the only vacant table. That showed his confidence in getting us out as quickly as he did.

I can't remember what I ate – not only was it a long time ago, but I was still a bag of nerves. I do know that the two men had steaks and I remember feeling quite nauseated when I saw the rareness of the meat, the blood oozing onto the plates.

After our plates were taken away, Pete's solicitor, who I now knew was called Jeremy, ordered cheese and biscuits to be served with a pot of coffee.

'You've a bit more colour in your face now, Amy, and I only have a few questions to ask you so nothing to worry about,' he told me.

I thought there was surely plenty to worry about, of which he was no doubt aware.

The first question that came my way was, 'Did they ask you anything about the car after they pulled you out of it?'

'No, they didn't mention anything about it when we were in the station,' I answered.

'And did they ask anything about your parents?'

'No. It was me, just before they told the constable to take me to the cell – I told them Mum was dead.'

'I know, Amy, and I'm truly sorry to hear it. You're certainly a brave girl. So, when you told them that, did they ask where your father was and had you got his phone number?'

'No. They only asked where I was staying and I gave Mrs Turner's address, not mine.'

'And that was all? They must have known that you didn't live there and that you were just a visitor. And did they ask for the phone number of an adult they could call?'

'The constable did and so I gave her Mrs Turner's number, but I don't think anyone called her.'

'No, she would have messaged me if they had,' said Pete checking his phone again.

'They knew it was the wrong address!' I exclaimed as a memory of something they said flashed into my mind. That was when the larger one was losing his temper and told me that my dad didn't seem bothered about me. That if he was, he would have rung the station to say I hadn't come home from school. Which means they knew all the time I lived with him.'

'Of course they did. One of the first questions they asked was where you lived. I told them the name of the village but said I hadn't got your address, but I knew you lived with your dad. They asked if that was because of a divorce or separation, so I told them that it wasn't, it was because your mother had died not that long ago.' Pete's words stunned me. For a few seconds, there was silence. I was shaking again at the thought of the police officers' cruelty. They had known all along that my mother was dead and that's why they said my dad and not my mum had not rung the station. And I know they never told the constable the truth either before she interviewed me. She was quite upset when I told them about losing Mum. Just reliving that part of the day almost made me burst into tears again, but I used every bit of determination not to.

'Sounds like they knew and yet they used the information to goad you. Despicable men, those two – they really shouldn't be in the force.'

I could tell by his expression that he was furious that an underage girl who had lost her mother had been treated in this way.

'So, if they knew all along that I had given them the wrong address, why didn't they ask for Dad's phone number?' I asked Jeremy.

'That's easy to work out,' he told me. 'They didn't want a concerned parent walking in, one who probably knew the basic laws surrounding interviewing children. It was Pete they were after, not you, and they wanted you to tell them something about him that they could use against him.'

The solicitor didn't ask me any more questions, which surprised me and I felt that he was being protective of me. He must have had a good idea of why they had made me feel so scared of them. They believed I was being stubborn in not giving them the information they wanted and they never considered that I might have been telling them the truth, or at least some of it.

Not being asked any more came as a relief – I hardly wanted to tell Jeremy about the threat of a police doctor giving me an intimate examination. Now I can guess that he knew exactly what the police were trying to prove. He had almost certainly asked Pete if there was anything I could tell them that could cause him a problem and, if there was, he'd better let him know. In fact, there was little he could have told Jeremy then. If only they had waited a day later, things might have been different.

'Are you going to make a complaint?' Pete wanted to know.

'If I do pursue the fact that Amy's father was not contacted, they will wave that piece of paper with their proof that she gave them the wrong address. And as for your friend Jacqui, everyone knows she's the local drunk and allows underage drinking in her home. Shame really because she's not a bad person. But that would give the police the perfect excuse. All they have to say is they phoned her and got no reply because she was probably out cold or just too drunk to answer. But they should have waited until I arrived before they questioned you, Amy,' said Jeremy.

'But they asked me loads,' I said indignantly.

'Your word against theirs, unfortunately.

Now, I can tell you're tired, Amy. I can drive you home. Don't think you're up to catching a bus.'

'Oh, don't worry,' said Pete quickly, 'I've already promised to do that.'

I noticed a kind of warning glance shooting in his direction from the solicitor. 'If you're sure you're up to it, Pete.'

'After eating that meal, I am,' he insisted.

'All right then, I'll take you back to where the car's parked. For once, those policemen did something sensible and parked it properly when they stopped you.'

'I'm surprised they did that,' said Pete. 'Must be about the only right thing they did.'

'They knew what would happen if the car was crashed into. Good thing the road you left it on wasn't a busy one. Made it easier for them to pull it over.'

'Thank you, Jeremy,' Pete said as we pulled up to where the car was parked. 'I'll take her home now.'

I glanced at him and he looked over at me and smiled.

Did he mean what he just said? I wondered. *I can only hope he doesn't.*

'Goodbye, Amy,' the solicitor said. 'I'm sorry you had such a horrid time there. It won't happen again, will it, Pete?'

'No, Jeremy, of course it won't.'

'Well, drive safely, your little friend needs to get home to sleep in her own bed.'

From the tone of his voice I knew that he was telling Pete to do just that. I learnt, not much later, that Jeremy was concerned about me mixing with Pete – but then he knew a lot more about him than I did.

'Don't worry, I'll be careful,' Pete told him.

We both thanked him for his time and the meal and then climbed into the car.

Pete waited for a few seconds until Jeremy's car had

disappeared from view before turning to me.

'I'm so sorry about what those policemen did to you. Do you still want to stay over at mine or shall I take you home?' he asked, placing an arm round my shoulders.

If only I had said home, but eager to please, I immediately said I would go to his.

'How are you feeling now?' he asked as he started the car.

'I'm all right,' I said – but I wasn't really. My head was throbbing and I felt completely worn out. All I really wanted to do was lie down on something comfortable, close my eyes and listen to that dreamy music of his.

We got to his parents' house in no time at all. Without any lights on it looked different, almost eerie. 'Let's get in quickly,' he said as, with his arm around me, we walked up to the door. He pulled the keys out of his pocket, quickly unlocked the door and switched on the lights.

'Are you OK climbing the stairs, Amy?'

'I think so,' I said as his concern made me smile. 'Doubt you want to piggyback me. I'll follow you so you can get the lights on up there.'

Walking into darkness after being in that dimly lit cell was not something I wanted to do. I felt a little better when, almost staggering into his room, it looked so peaceful and comfy.

'You get on that bed and relax. There's plenty of pillows to prop you up while I get us both a drink. I expect you could do with one. I know I could, seeing as we only had fizzy water with dinner."

I nodded and got onto the bed. He was right: after lying for so long on that hard wooden bench with its skimpy mattress, it felt so soft and cosy. I pulled my arms up over my head and stretched as hard as I could. Pete plumped up some more pillows and placed them behind my head so that I could sit up. The music I liked came on more or less the same time as a glass of wine was placed in my hand. It only took a few sips for me to begin to feel every part of me relaxing. Up until then I had been so tense, I was aching all over.

Pete sat on the chair by the bed and it was not long before a second glass of wine was poured. He clearly wanted to know what the police had asked, especially as I had blushed when Jeremy was probing me.

'Did they ask you if I was your boyfriend?'

'They didn't ask; they kept telling me they knew you were.'

'And what did you say?'

'That you were just a friend and then the big one said you were too old to be that.'

'What was your answer?'

'That you were one of the older people who looked out for me because my mother was dead. He pretended not to know. I can't believe they already knew that.'

'Bastards, aren't they, those two? It was brave of you to bring that up. I know how upsetting that must have been,' and he leant over and hugged me. 'It was so good of you to tell them about your mum. It makes me feel guilty that they used you like that to get at me.

'I was worried about you when I was in my cell but I knew you wouldn't say anything that would get me in trouble. I just hoped you knew that part of the law, but you do, don't you?'

'Yes, the law says we're not allowed to sleep together because I'm not yet sixteen and you're eighteen.'

'What a stupid law that is, don't you think? I try and do everything that makes you happy and they would love to put me in prison if they thought you and I were a couple. And we are, aren't we?'

That made me feel warm and loved.

'As long as I don't end up in that police station again,' I said, which made him laugh. He didn't seem to realise then that I wasn't joking. I stopped myself from saying, 'It's more than only sleeping together that they accused me of.' I didn't want to talk about what happened anymore. In the whole of my young life, adults had always been kind to me. I never could have imagined being treated that way and I had been, and still was, shaken by it. Images of how my home life had once been, when I never felt anything but safe and loved, caused tears to form in my eyes – I just wanted him to hold me, stroke my back and comfort me.

All these thoughts were tumbling around in my head and it made me not want to talk about us going further than we already had. So far, we were not really breaking any laws. Besides, I still wasn't sure I wanted to do more. Other girls at school were starting to talk about what they did with boys, but he was the first one that I had ever really talked to, let alone kissed.

I didn't want to say to him that they were trying to make me admit I had sex with him. Either they didn't believe me, or they thought they could intimidate me enough to say what they wanted. The way they treated me made me feel that they saw me as a despicable youngster. Not only that, but I had also felt that Jeremy believed that I was not only a young friend of Pete's that he was giving a lift to. Did he also think we were having sex? I could tell by the way he had said I needed to get home and into my own bed that he was sending some kind of message to Pete, a message he promptly ignored.

I was happy enough then not to mind that he had. But it took only a few months for me to have wished he had listened to Jeremy.

It was while the music played that the joints got rolled. Drawing up that dope didn't have a good effect on me at all. Instead, it made me feel even more tired.

I told him that my headache was still there.

'I can see you're very pale,' Pete said as he looked up at my face. 'I think you're still upset about today, and who wouldn't be?'

'Maybe too much wine and smoking dope at the same time has made it worse,' I suggested.

'I have something that will make you feel better. Shall I give it to you?' he offered.

As I was fairly stoned by then I didn't think to ask what it was he was offering me and so I nodded.

'It's just a little something, it will make you feel much better and more relaxed straight away.'

But I still didn't ask what it was or what he was doing. Stupidly, I trusted him and anything that would make me feel better had to be worth having. I know now exactly what it was he was busy mixing: a white powder – a mix of citric acid and water – was placed on a spoon, then he flicked his lighter underneath until it was fully dissolved. What did I do? I sat on the bed and watched. I didn't know that was to be the moment when years of my life were to be destroyed. If only time travelling was real and not fiction, I would go back to that exact second, ask what it was, then say no and insist that I wanted to go home. How I wish I had stopped him. Unfortunately, I wasn't up to questioning anything and so I just did what Pete told me: I rolled up my sleeve so that he could tie a shoelace around my arm. That, I soon learnt, was to make a vein stand out enough to insert a needle.

I might have been stoned, but I can still remember clearly how I looked at the walls of the room while Tracy Chapman's 'Fast Car' was playing in the background. Even now I can feel that sharp scratch and the stinging feeling in my arm as the drug travelled up the vein. Within seconds it turned my depression and tension into ecstasy. The lace on my arm came loose and I fell back on the pillows. All my fear, all the pain of my memories, vanished. I wished I could feel that way forever.

I'll never forget how I woke up sneezing, sweating and shaking. My first thought was that it must be the flu, but it was the words that came out of Pete's mouth that I was naive enough to believe that damaged my life forever.

'Amy, I'm so sorry!'

'Why? What... you sorry for?' I murmured.

Without answering, he took hold of the pencil case again and went through the process again, then grasped my arm, peered down at the veins in it and quickly injected me. Almost straight away, the pain, the shaking and the sweating ceased. I felt good again and fell back on the bed. Within what seemed like seconds, I drifted off to my new world: the place where everything was all right and nothing else mattered. Then I heard the words, 'I'm so sorry, Amy, I've given you a habit. You're going to need these injections fairly regularly.'

I know now that Pete was not at all sorry. It was only when I met other addicts that I learnt why I had sweated and shook so much: he had mixed the heroin with crack cocaine. He waited for the effect on me to happen and then gave me another injection that stopped it. All this he used to make me reliant on him. Of course, I know now that had been his intention all along. I can never understand how he felt so much for my teenage self that he would have done anything to keep me with him. He would have said it was love but that's not love, is it? He destroyed my life and his only excuse was that he worshipped the ground I walked on.

Now you can see why I wanted to rip out some of those pages in my younger self's diary. I would never write about my feelings in my diary again.

Only notes to remind me of something.

Which is the same reason I never got rid of them. There were certain days when it might have been better to forget but I chose not to.

That was the punishment I gave to myself.

19

That weekend with Pete is another memory that I would like to erase from my mind but, instead, I decided to keep the pictures of that time firmly embedded. Why, Amy? You might well ask this question. The answer is that I have a teenage daughter. What mother with a past like mine would not worry just how easily young people can be tempted to experiment with drugs? I can only wish that teenagers come to realise how much harm drugs can do to their bodies in only a few years. Oh, we can think that as responsible parents we're keeping an eye on them and are reassured when we meet their friends that they're mixing with the right people. If only it were that simple.

Pete came from a well-off family and he spoke with an educated accent; he was also extremely good-looking and charming. Just the type that mothers might approve of. When a picture of him flies into my head, I almost shudder with revulsion. He used every trick in the book to make me infatuated with him. In his twisted mind, he had decided that, once I was dependant on him, I would never walk away.

It took me a while to realise exactly what he had done. That night, after I had been in the cell, I was in no state to question why he wanted to inject me. Even worse, I didn't ask him what would be in that syringe. OK, I know now that he lied repeatedly, so even if I had asked, he would have done it again. It's a shame that at that age I was totally unaware of how dangerous it was to agree to have a non-medical person inject me.

Going back to that day, I can almost hear him saying, 'I'm so sorry, Amy, I've given you a habit' – 'habit' meaning thanks to him I was addicted. Just hearing that sentence in my head makes me feel sick with anger. And if that was forgivable – which I don't think it is – his next little piece of giving me what he called 'the facts' was not. Again, I can hear his smooth voice telling me why I was going to have to come to him regularly to have an injection because, if I didn't, I would be much sicker than I had been that first time – 'You could end up in hospital, Amy, and you don't want that to happen, do you?'

'No, I don't,' I said shakily as I remembered how Mum had died in one. That was enough to make me even more frightened. I believed every word he told me then. All these years later, I have never been able to forgive him. How could he have mixed the drugs to make me feel so ill? What I worked out a long time ago was that so much of what he did was planned. Was he the one who made sure the police would be waiting for us when we left Jacqui's? Just one phone call would have done that and disguising his voice a little was something he was good at. That suspicion is something I have never found proof of, but it's still something I believe he did.

I wish the police, instead of trying get me to admit I was having sex with Pete, had talked about the dangers of taking drugs. Didn't they think pushing heroin into an underage girl's arm was even worse than persuading her to have sex with him? They knew that he and Dave both took and sold drugs, but it was just one of the things they had not been able to catch them doing.

Still, I can almost feel the fear and panic I went through as Pete told me that I was now an addict sunk in. He made sure that, before I left his home, I believed that the only way I could remain healthy was to go to him for injections on a regular basis. Didn't I realise that after twenty-four hours when the drug had left my body, I would be all right?

The fact is, I didn't. I knew nothing about drugs and back then there was nothing on the topic in our school curriculum, certainly not for my year. Pete had drummed into my head that, if I left it more than six days, my next bout of illness would be far worse than the first one. The only excuse I have for believing that nonsense was that I was still very young and naive.

As I left Pete's house and headed home, I realised it was only two weeks away from my birthday. Naturally, over the next few days I wondered what Dad was going to arrange for me. Apart from the money he gave me to buy whatever it was I wanted, nothing much had been done about birthdays or Christmas since Mum's death. Having got used to that,

I wasn't expecting much to happen. The only good thing I had been told about was that Janet was coming for a few days and, even better, my aunt was staying with us. I supposed Dad would take us out for an evening meal and invite Anne and her family to come too.

I had to tell Pete that my aunt was coming to see me and that the day would just be a family thing so I couldn't go out with him on my birthday.

'Aren't you having a party and then you could invite me?' he said.

'I don't think so.'

Even then, I was becoming aware that I was living two lives. There were the people I knew at Jacqui's and the teenagers in our village. Mixing them together would not have been a good idea. And the niggling worry I was trying to cope with was that everyone would see something about me that would tell them I was an addict. I didn't have a clue then that it took a lot longer than having only two hits in one day for it to become evident.

Pete put his arm around me when I asked him about this and said, 'Of course they wouldn't think that. All they would say is how much better you're looking since the last time they saw you. And you do. When you look in the mirror, you'll know I'm right.'

20

I can remember almost all my birthdays. There are some that I wish I couldn't. In a way, my thirteenth birthday is one of them.

It turned out to be the last one that my family would ever arrange. I still had some of my childhood innocence left then, but a year later not one member of my family thought of me in the same way.

When I look back at some of the notes I wrote a long time ago, it takes my mind back to the days of earlier childhood birthday parties. Each year when Mum was still there, she must have spent a lot of time arranging them because they were all really special. After she died, I don't think my father gave them much thought. I was given money to buy whatever I wanted and I was taken out by Aunt Janet, who always appeared around then, and we once went with Dad to the family night at the club. But birthdays were no longer a joyous occasion for me as they just made me miss Mum even more. When I think of all the effort she put into my birthday parties, it almost makes me cry. She even had one for my first birthday, and no, I can't remember that. I have seen the photos, though, which show how happy the three of us were.

I'm not going to write pages about all the parties Mum arranged, but I would like to tell you about the last one she gave me. She was full of fun that day. A couple of days earlier, Dad had bought a BBQ. 'Look,' he told us, carrying the huge box into the garden shed, 'we can use that on your birthday, Amy, and I'll be King of the Grill!' Mum and I laughed because we knew who would be in the kitchen for hours before making salads, marinades and the cake. That BBQ was another item that never got used again after Mum's death.

Mum told me it would only be a family gathering this time, except, of course, for her friend Anne and her sons, but they were like family. Dad was going to take me with him to fetch Gran, his mother, who I adored. Even so, that didn't stop me from feeling a little disappointed that my friends wouldn't be there.

It was quite a long drive to where Gran lived. I sat in the car with my seat belt firmly on, looking out of the window. As we drove through the country lanes leading to Gran's cottage, I could see masses of wildflowers in the hedgerows and in the fields behind them were cows with their cute little calves, which I kept pointing out to Dad. A few minutes later, we pulled up outside Gran's house. We had hardly reached the door before it opened and she stepped out. Frail as she appeared then, her smile was still a sparkling one. Her arms must have kept strong with all the gardening she did because, when she gave me a huge hug, I could feel they were far from weak. She picked up the bag she had brought to the door but Dad took it gently from her and popped it into the boot of the car. He then helped her into the front seat while I retreated to the back.

Gran must have known exactly what the arrangements were, for when, about three quarters of an hour later, we walked into the kitchen, I heard the word 'surprise' being shouted by at least ten of my closest friends.

The cake Mum had made for me looked like a dark wooden cottage with a roof of white icing. She had also covered the ground around it in the same colour icing to make it look like snow. In front of the cottage were the words 'Happy Birthday' and a tiny figure of a girl was positioned in the middle of those words.

I don't think I've ever seen a cake as beautiful as that one.

When I saw the pile of presents on the table, I gasped a little.

'Better start opening them,' Mum told me.

At that young age I didn't need any persuasion. My eager fingers could hardly wait to open them up. I can't remember all the presents I was given but I do know there were pretty hair slides and an Alice band, a book or two and a pink beaded necklace. Gran had given me a pale yellow jumper and the present from my parents, which I had been given that morning, was a tiny gold locket on a chain. I had seen it in the jewellery shop and told Mum that I thought it was so lovely.

There were lots of games that we played out in the garden. Anne's two boys and I used the skipping rope first and then my other friends wanted their turn. Dad got the BBQ going and my uncles gathered by to chat as they waited for the flames to go down so that Dad could put the sausages on the grill. Once they were cooked, Mum put them in white rolls along with some sauce. 'Hot dogs,' she announced as, putting them on paper plates, she handed them out to the queue forming around her.

'Your mum's so cool,' sighed one of my friends.

'She is, she's the best mum ever,' I agreed with a happy grin.

That moment was captured on a photo that Dad took and I still have it today.

Once all the hot dogs had been eaten, Mum took hold of my hand and told everyone she was taking me in so we could cut the cake and soon everyone was back into the kitchen. Ten candles were lit, making the cake look even more pretty.

'You're going to have to blow them out and then make a wish, one that you're not to share with anyone. Remember, it's your secret and you must keep it for yourself,' Mum whispered to me.

So I drew as much air into my lungs as I could, leant down close to the candle flames and blew as hard as I could. Out they all went, making everyone cheer me, and then they all sang 'Happy Birthday'. Mum got busy slicing the cake into generous pieces, which everyone said was delicious. And it was, I assure you. I should think everyone was full by the time they left later in the afternoon. Aunt Janet was staying with us and Anne and her family stayed on a little longer too. Dad brought out wine, while Mum got tea for Gran and cola for me and Anne's sons.

I know I was pretty tired when Mum helped me carry all my gifts upstairs. Then I quickly washed and brushed my teeth before getting into pyjamas and bed. Mum tucked me in, kissed me goodnight and, after leaving the door a little open, she went back downstairs. I think I had already fallen fast asleep before she got to the bottom.

21

We had a free paper in Normanton called *The Advertiser*. On the back of it were the notices of births, marriages, deaths, anniversaries, funeral announcements and, of course, special birthdays. I can understand the wedding and birthday announcements, but not deaths. I mean, who wants to be reminded of something heartbreaking every year?

One day, I popped into a shop on the way to school to pick up a cool drink and I remember seeing the following announcement:

Remembering Mary Pearson, 41, who passed away peacefully at Pinderfields Hospital. Her funeral was held at Pontefract Crematorium on 2 April 1996. The much-loved wife of John and a loving mum to her only daughter, Amy-Jayne. She is sadly missed by her family and her many friends.

Just what I wanted to read on what was my thirteenth birthday. That piece in the newspaper brought back the image in my head of how Mum had looked the last time I saw her in hospital. She was far from peaceful then, which had upset me and angered Dad so much that we left the ward as fast as possible.

How I wished I hadn't seen that paper so early in the day. I suppose whoever wrote it and placed it in the paper didn't think that it might spoil my birthday. As I walked to school, I crossed my fingers, hoping the day would go all right. The pupils in my class and some of those in the senior classes that I was friendly with knew that it was my birthday and I just hoped there wouldn't be any jokey pranks coming in my direction. Both that paper and my so-called 'need for drugs' had left me rather depressed but, that morning, it soon turned out that I needn't have worried about any jokes. As I walked through the gates, I heard a chorus of 'Happy birthday, Amy.' That, as well as the hugs and pats on my shoulders as quite a few of my classmates crowded round me, took my mind off the newspaper and put a smile on my face.

There were so many cards pushed into my hands that I hardly knew where to put them.

'There's something on your desk inside,' my close friend Maddy told me and I could tell by her face that she thought it might be a joke of some kind. Thankfully, it wasn't. Talk about being surprised! I looked at my desk and propped up on top was a huge card with an old junior school photo of me with the words, 'Happy 13th Birthday, Amy-Jayne. You're a Teenager Now! Your mum would be so proud of you. All my love, Dad'.

If that amazed me, the thirteen kisses on it astounded me.

To me, this was so special and I forgot that most days we barely spoke. I pictured my father going through all our family photos until he found this one. Then he would have taken it to the printer to have it enlarged and turned into that wonderful card. I was so touched that I had to wipe away the tears that came into my eyes. Throughout the day I kept the card on my desk and, as we changed classrooms for our different lessons, it went with me – I couldn't stop glancing at it every few seconds.

There was another surprise for me when school finished: Dad was waiting in his car outside the school gate. It was a good thing that Pete hadn't turned up to give me a present, even though I had told him I had to go straight home. What a relief – this was not the day for them to meet and I would have had a lot of explaining to do.

'Jump in, Amy,' said Dad as he pushed the door open for me and I did as quickly as possible. There were a few people I didn't want him to meet or, more to the point, hear them call out something like, 'Aren't you coming to Jacqui's? It's your birthday, let's get a bit pissed there.' As far as he knew, not a drop of alcohol had ever passed my lips.

When he announced that he would be taking me shopping in Wakefield, I was a little taken aback: 'I decided it would be better if you choose what you want for your birthday,' he said. I could hardly believe what I was hearing. Usually he gave me money and told me to go shopping with Anne.

'There's one shop I want you to take a look in,' he told me as we drove into Wakefield and he pulled up in front of a jewellery shop. 'I saw something in there that in your language is supposed to be trendy,' he said with an almost mischievous smile as he pointed to a ring chain. My eyes widened when I looked at it. What could be cooler than having a chain going from my finger to my wrist? Beaming with pleasure, I turned to him.

'I love it, Dad,' I told him.

'Then let's go inside and get it, Amy.'

Dad told the man behind the counter what it was he wanted me to try on. The ring chain fitted perfectly. I didn't want to take it off and told him so.

'Then you don't have to. You can have the box to keep it in because there's no way you can wear something like that to school,' he cautioned.

Tucking the box in my satchel while Dad paid, I was glowing with happiness. When the pair of us walked back to the car, I kept looking down at my hand as my silver ring chain sparkled on it.

I expected that we would be going back home then, but no, he drove a little further into town, parked the car next to a meter and dropped a couple of coins into it.

'I think you need something that will set off your ring chain well,' was all he said.

I stopped myself asking just when he had found out the name of the shop that was full of fashionable teenage clothes. One look at the selection of clothes in the window was enough to tell me that it was going to be full of them. If that surprised me, so did the fact that he came in, sat down on a chair near the dressing room and told me to start looking for what I wanted.

On hearing him, the shop assistant smiled and came over to us and asked me what it was I was looking for.

'An outfit that will show this off,' I said, waving the hand with my ring chain on it in front of her.

We ran through a few things until I chose a pair of black jeans with silver studs on the back pockets. They were a definite, but I couldn't decide between a white shirt and a white cotton jumper with single silver threading on the bottom. Putting on first one and then the other, I went out of the changing room each time and asked Dad which one suited me the most.

'Have them both, they look great on you,' he told me as he took out his credit card for the second time that day.

I was so pleased by his compliments that my cheeks burned. The way he was that day made me feel that he was just like my dad in the old days.

'Better get home quickly, your aunt will be waiting for us,' he said after he had paid and everything had been wrapped up for me.

I was really happy to see my Aunt Janet waiting for us when we walked in. She was someone I always missed when she went back to her home and she looked as cheerful as I was feeling that day.

'Here's a little something for you,' she told me, handing me a large envelope and a small pink parcel.

I opened the envelope first. Inside was a birthday card with such fond greetings from Janet and her family that it made me throw my arms around her.

'You'd better open the parcel, Amy,' Dad said. 'You might think what's inside is even better than the card.'

I took his advice gleefully and gasped with pleasure when I saw what it was: a velvet-lined box with a silver necklace inside. Dad must have told my aunt what he had in mind for me because her present went so well with my dainty ring chain.

This was certainly a birthday I was enjoying. It was once we were in the kitchen having cups of tea that I realised it was far from over when Dad told me we would celebrate my birthday at the club – 'Anne and her family plus a few other people will be joining us, so when you've finished that tea, off you go and get yourself ready. Wear that new outfit of yours!'

Getting ready took me a little time – after all, I was now officially a teenager. Hair washed and blow-dried, the tiniest amount of make-up applied and then a wriggle into my new black jeans and white shirt. The jumper went around my shoulders and my new necklace and ring chain completed the look. As I stood in front of the mirror, admiring my new outfit and my silver jewellery, I had a feeling that it was going to be a good night. I hadn't seen Dad looking so cheerful or heard him praise me in such a long time. It was that which made me smile so happily at my reflection.

More compliments came my way when I went downstairs. Dad had changed into a suit and Janet looked pretty in the dress she had chosen to wear as well.

'Time to go,' said Dad as he looked at his watch. 'Don't want to keep people waiting. We can get something to eat there.'

I could hardly believe what I saw when we walked in. There must have been over thirty people waiting for us as we arrived.

Being on the club's committee meant that Dad had managed to do a lot more than I was expecting. When he had said we could get something to eat there, he really meant it.

Judging by the amount of food on the long table, he and Janet had been busy planning the party. There was a huge birthday cake, platters and dishes piled high with all kinds of food, sweet and savoury. There was even some bunting on the wall with the words 'Happy Birthday, Amy' on it.

There were more cards and quite a few parcels and gift bags. Dad told everyone that he would put them in the car and I would open them later – 'She might as well let her birthday carry on until breakfast time!' he said and everyone laughed.

Dad allowed me to have one glass of bubbly. I liked the bubbles, although I had to pretend that I had never tasted alcohol before.

Yes, it was a great evening.

So, if it was all so great, why did I write earlier that it was a birthday I wanted to forget?

The answer is that within a few weeks I felt that everything Dad had arranged and paid for was acts of bribery, not love.

22

It didn't take long after Janet had left for Dad to change from the caring father back to the one that I had been living with since Mum died. Not that I noticed straight away because he still seemed pretty cheerful. It all changed for me when a few days later he announced that he was going to Thailand. I should have known that was the reason he was in such an elated mood – I could hardly believe that it had just been planned so he waited to tell me after my birthday.

For a few moments I felt a tinge of excitement as I waited for the magic words that he would be taking me there with him. He knew how much I loved seeing different countries and it sounded so wonderful. When I thought how many places we had visited when Mum was alive, I hadn't understood why he had stopped taking me with him since our trip to Turkey. As it was nearly the school holidays, there was no reason for me not to go with him, so I waited patiently for him to say what I hoped to hear.

My heart sank when I realised that he wasn't going to ask me to go with him. I knew he had liked Thailand ever since he first went off on a boys-only holidays with his close friend Joe and a couple of other pals. That had just been a short trip. When he went the first time, I didn't really care – I was happy enough staying with Anne when he was away. The second time I was a little older and I had heard the rumours of why single men go over to Thailand, but I just shrugged my shoulders when some of the girls told me that this when I mentioned Dad was there.

I suppose he can do what he wants to, I made myself think, even though I hardly liked what I had heard.

But the trip just after my birthday had a very different effect on me. From the moment I had seen that card on my desk and been thrilled by everything my father had done for me, I believed that he still loved me, even though I had doubted it for quite a while. Since Mum had died, there had been so many occasions when I felt that he did his best to avoid spending time with me. When she was still with us, I had always felt that I was loved by both my parents. I knew he had cared for me when I was younger and there had been the occasional act of kindness over the last three years. Since that great party he had organised and the presents he had given me, I felt we were now on a new footing and so I started to imagine us going out together more often. Like having a meal out or going with him to the club on family days. All that had stopped, but that didn't mean I couldn't hope it would start again. I almost dreamt of coming home from school to hear his voice calling out my name. So, there I was, still with the remnants of hope in my heart, even though I already knew what he was going to say.

I think you can guess how I felt when, looking me in the eye, he said, 'I've arranged for you to stay with Anne. I know you like it there.'

Yes, I did, but I also loved travelling to different countries like we did when Mum was alive. I was about to blurt that out but luckily that sensible inner voice of mine told me not to.

The reward for my silence was a wad of notes that he handed to me. Then came some caring words, which hardly impressed me: 'I know you like going out with your friends and I'm pretty sure that you might miss the bus so there's enough for taxis there and whatever you need to spend when you are out. I've already given Anne enough cash to cover your food and your share of the electricity. Oh, and Amy, if you plan to stay over with some of your friends, make sure you let her know well before – you don't want her cooking for you if you're not going to be in, do you?'

There was no way then that I couldn't help but feel that all the kindness he had shown me was to get me on side so he could get up to who knows what while he was away. It didn't take long for him to convince me that my suspicions were totally correct. He'd told both Anne and I that he would be away for a fortnight. I was at school when he called Anne to say that he was staying on for another fortnight. He didn't tell her the reason then – I expect she just thought that he must be having a good time, but all Anne told me was that he was staying on for another couple of weeks. I didn't realise it at the time but soon realised that my dad had also quit his job.

Another call came after a week, telling her the date that he was going to arrive. His two weeks away had turned into six. I would be back at school by the time he came back.

I could tell by the way that Anne could hardly look me in the face that he had told her something upsetting.

'Why? What is it, Anne?' I asked.

'Oh, he'll be back soon and he can explain everything to you then. He's ringing you later, just try not to get angry with him,' she advised. 'At least he has sent money to my bank, which is for both of us. There's another fifty that he asked me to give you.'

'That's good of him,' I said sarcastically before going up-stairs to change out of my uniform. This was an evening that I was to be staying in – I didn't want to annoy Anne by being out all the time. She must have already sensed that other things were going on, how could she not?

Just as I was wondering how I could get her to tell me what was going on over in Thailand, the phone rang. I don't know why, but I guessed it was Dad ringing.

Better go down, I told myself.

I was right, it was Dad on the phone. As I walked down the stairs, I heard Anne say, 'Maybe you'd better leave telling her until you get back home, John.'

I think he might have argued that he had every right to speak to me then.

She looked up and saw me. 'It's your dad. He wants to speak to you,' she said with her hand over the receiver. 'He's got something to tell you. Don't let him upset you,' she added before passing me the phone and walked quickly back into the kitchen, closing the door behind her to give me some privacy.

What he told me was beyond anything that had entered my imagination. His first sentence was that he had married a Thai woman and that he hoped to bring her back to England. I must have shouted something like, 'I don't want to hear anything more,' because Anne came rushing up just as I slammed the phone down.

'Careful not to break it, love' she said, looking worried.

'It's his neck I'd like to break. How could he do that, and never mention it to me?' I said.

'I can see that you've had a bit of a shock. Come into the kitchen and we can talk, Amy.'

The kettle had already boiled – she must have known what my reaction was going to be and it was easier to talk to me with a cup in her hand.

'Look, Amy,' she said once we were sitting down, 'he'll be back soon. You can talk to him then. I know your dad really loved your mum and, from what I saw, he was heartbroken after her death. And yes, I know you were too. Like you, he's missed her a lot and I suppose he wanted someone he could be close to again so try and understand that a little.'

But I couldn't, not then. It was all a total shock to me and, hard as I tried not to, I burst into tears.

'How could he?' I kept saying. 'Why didn't he tell me before he left and why didn't he want me at the wedding?'

'That I don't know,' said Anne.

'Is he bringing her back with him? I don't want to live in a house with his new wife. I couldn't stand it – sleeping in Mum's bed and bossing me about.'

'Let's just wait and see what happens,' she said as she put her arm round me in an effort to calm me down.

I could tell, even though she tried not to show it, that she was disgusted with him. Wanting to marry again was not strange for a widower of his age but doing it so quickly, keeping quiet about it and not letting his friends or his daughter know was, to her mind, bang out of order.

When he did come back to England, thankfully, he was alone.

23

Between Dad arriving home and then leaving me again, I went off the rails. I would say that's the most accurate description of my behaviour and actions at that time.

It was after that phone call that my resentment came to a head. Did he think I would cheerfully go along with everything he did? The sad thing was that, over the three years since Mum had died, I had managed to cope with his lack of affection towards me. Now, when I go back in time, I recognise that my coping strategy with him faded after that phone call. Faded, but not completely disappeared. I still wanted to cling to how, on my birthday, he had gone back to his old self – the father who was more than fond of me. Beside my bed was the card with its thirteen kisses on it, though it didn't take me too long to tear into pieces.

Up until the day he arrived back from Thailand, there remained a small spark of hope inside that he would want to apologise for not telling me sooner that he had met someone, a woman he had decided to marry. Maybe then I would have had time to process the news and accept her. I knew the time and the day the plane was due, but neither Anne nor I had been told if he was coming straight back to our home or not.

'Most likely Joe will pick him up and those two could well go somewhere for a drink,' I said as I remembered the pair of them knocking back cans of beer when Joe picked us up on the day we returned from Turkey.

'Oh, I don't think he'll waste much time. I expect he'll want to explain a few things to you. No doubt he'll come here first and take you back to the house,' said Anne. 'You'd better have your stuff all packed – you don't want to keep him waiting.'

So I did as she suggested and packed everything into my suitcase, apart from a change of clothes that I could put on when I came back from school.

Once I knew the time that the plane would be landing, I felt nervous but not as tense and worried as I was on the day he was arriving. After all, I had slammed the phone down on him, which was enough to make him angry. I knew he was arriving on his own because he had already said that his new wife had some visa problems.

I kept asking myself what he would be like with me now that he had remarried. Anne had told me to come straight back from school and I rushed out of the gates, not stopping to chat with anyone, and ran as fast as I could to the bus stop so that I could catch an earlier one than usual. I managed to get there just as the bus drew up. Anne's boys and some of their friends were going to play football and would catch the later bus. As her husband didn't get back from work until around six, it would be just Anne and me in the house when Dad arrived.

As I walked to Anne's from where the bus had dropped me off, I wondered if Dad would already be there.

'He's not phoned yet to say where he is,' Anne told me as soon as I dumped my satchel in the hall and followed her into the kitchen. I must have been halfway through my cup of tea when the phone rang and she rushed to answer it.

I heard her say Dad's name in a friendly way and then her tone of voice changed. Whatever he was saying wasn't pleasing her. More than once I heard, 'But John...' It was obvious to me that he wouldn't let her finish her sentence. I don't know what it was he was saying, only that it was enough to make her annoyed.

'Is he on his way?' I asked when she came back.

'He's already at the house and he wants you to walk over there now. He told me to tell you not to take anything with you, he's not staying there long,' she sighed.

'What else did he say?'

Judging by the length of the call, he had said more than that.

'Not much really, just that he had to sort out a few things with you.'

I could guess what they were. Still, I didn't have much choice but to go home and face him. I could tell that Anne was worried. She had seen how devastated I was when Mum died, having a breakdown when the ball of grief hit me. I had finally turned a corner when she had witnessed me so full of happiness at my thirteenth birthday party. She was also aware of how much my dad had neglected me over almost three years. I'm sure that, after what he had just said to her, she was even more concerned about the impact of his behaviour on me.

'I can drive you there if you like,' she offered.

'Thanks, but I'm all right walking there. I could do with some fresh air. It might clear my head.'

Not that an intake of fresh air helped because I was still a bundle of nerves when I reached the house I had always thought of as home. I hesitated, trying to make up my mind whether to just walk in or ring the bell. As I hovered on the doorstep, Dad opened the door and told me to come in.

With his deep suntan and his short-sleeved T-shirt that showed a new tattoo on his arm, he looked different to me.

'Let's go into the kitchen. I've made a pot of coffee so we can talk at the table,' he said.

His tone of voice made me even more nervous – it was as though he was talking to a complete stranger, not his teenage daughter. And it didn't take long for me to feel that it was me who was talking to a different person. The one thing I noticed when he poured out the coffee was that there was no smell of drink on him. Now that was little unusual because normally he would have been holding a can of beer to his lips.

'Look, Amy,' he said as he sat down opposite me, 'if we're ever going to spend some time together, you have to accept that you now have a new mother. She's sent you a present, which I don't think you deserve, but I'll give it to you anyway.'

How I seethed. I wanted to scream and shout at him. Even if he wanted a new wife, I didn't want a new mother. Sitting there, looking at the father who hadn't once smiled at me since I entered the house, made me feel far too uptight to say anything. Any courage I might have had deserted me.

Seeing that I was not going to say anything negative about his wife, Dad bent down and pulled out a large paper carrier from under the table, handing it to me.

'Her present for you is inside,' he told me, his voice quite cold, almost indifferent.

I pushed my hand in and drew out a turquoise silk scarf. Yes, it was pretty, but I didn't want it. Had he told me that it was from both of them, I might have been slightly more pleased. Still, I managed to say thank you.

'I'll tell her you liked it,' he said. 'Now tell me why you slammed the phone down on me.'

If only he had let that go, then I wouldn't have blurted out, 'Because you never told me anything about your being involved with her, or that you were going to marry her. I don't want a new mother, I'm still missing Mum. I still see her in my head whenever I'm here.' At least I managed not to say that I couldn't bear the thought of another woman walking around the house that was entirely furnished to Mum's taste.

He ignored the fact that I was clearly upset and just glared at me. 'I had hoped that my thoughts that you are just a jealous little girl weren't true. I can see now they are. You resent me having found someone who makes me happy and, if you cared, you would be pleased for me. But you're not. You've no right to feel that way. Until you've worked out that's wrong, you can stay at Anne's. You've said what you wanted to and now you can leave,' he told me.

I tried to say something, like how much I missed him, but I could tell he had no intention of listening to me.

'Amy, I've said leave now.'

Tears were splashing down my cheeks as I made it to the front door. Slamming it shut behind me, I ran as fast as I could back to Anne's. He must have phoned her the minute I left the house because she was waiting outside for me. Before I could say anything, she wrapped her arms round me while I sobbed my heart out.

'He doesn't want me to stay in the house with him,' I told her once I had managed to stop crying enough to speak.

'I know, dear, but we all love having you here. Your dad will come round, just you wait and see,' she told me gently. 'Now let's go in.'

She didn't say anything else about my father then, though no doubt she had plenty to say about his behaviour to her husband later.

'The boys will be back soon. I love them, but I think I would rather be in my room,' I said shakily.

Almost certainly, they would have some questions for me and Anne understood that I wouldn't want to talk about it. They knew that Dad was coming back and me not being in the house with him would make them curious.

'Yes, of course, Amy,' she agreed. 'I think it will be more peaceful for you to be in your room today. I'll bring your supper up later. The boys won't be back for a good half hour, so let's have a cup of tea and a piece of cake together before you go upstairs.'

Anne really did her best to cheer me up as we sat together

in the living room but I was so forlorn, I just wanted to be on my own. Just before the boys were due back, I went to my room and lay down on the bed. All I could think of once I was alone was how wonderful the years of my earlier childhood had been. Up until when Mum had been rushed into hospital, I'd have to say it was pretty perfect. Both my parents had shown me so much love – I couldn't have asked for anything more.

I now honestly believe that, if I'd been a boy, my relationship with my father might have been different. At thirteen, I didn't understand that every time he saw me, he loathed the fact that I looked so much like Mum. He must have wanted to push the hurt of losing her out of his mind. My dark hair and large brown eyes were so like hers, I suppose it was a permanent reminder of what he had lost. If that wasn't upsetting enough, despite being the daughter he loved, I'm convinced that my father never forgave me for being recognised by Mum at the hospital when he wasn't. Those last words he heard coming from her must have shaken him to the core. I've never forgotten that look of hatred on his face, a look that was directed at me.

That night, after he told me to get out of the house, I got more upset the more I thought about it. The expression on his face then was the same as the one in the hospital – the one I had tried so hard to forget. It was then that I knew I had lost both my parents.

Looking back, I can still feel a surge of anger at how he treated my younger self. How could he have worked so hard at making his daughter feel like an orphan? Even now some of those memories bring tears to my eyes. I can remember the time when I needed him the most, he wasn't there for me. Nor was he in the house that much. Little wonder I fell in with the wrong crowd. He seemed to think that handing me more money than I needed compensated for his lack of love towards me. He never showed any interest in what I did in my spare time or who my friends were.

Then on my thirteenth birthday, why did he bother? Did he pay someone at my school to put that card with thirteen kisses on it on my desk? That night, I ripped it into tiny pieces before tossing it in the bin and then I told myself to forget what he had done.

I had Pete and my other friends, didn't I?

* * *

Two days after I had been thrown out of what I was once my home, I told Anne that I would be spending the night with a friend. I needed some time with Pete and to see everyone at Jacqui's house as well.

'That will do you good,' she said.

It didn't.

What I really wanted was to spend the night with Pete. I could really do with some affection, which he would give me. I couldn't, though, because his parents were in the house and, although he was free to come and go, arriving with a thirteen-year-old girl who stayed the night would be impossible. The second choice was Jacqui's, who I phoned to ask if I could stay there.

'Come when you're ready,' she told me.

It would be easy to get smashed on cider there, but it was my drug that I needed more. I already knew that a hit would take away my misery. I was meeting Pete after school and I was pretty sure he would have it with him.

The boys and I walked together to the bus stop in the morning. Not one question was asked and I wondered what Anne must have told them. Whatever it was, Dad was not mentioned. Although I was determined not to let my unhappiness about Dad affect my schoolwork, I did find it hard to concentrate. At break times I tried to be my cheerful self and I think I managed that not too badly. As soon as school ended, I made a beeline for the toilets and quickly changed into my jeans and a baggy jumper before racing out of the gates.

I was so pleased when I found Pete standing just outside, waiting for me. He had only just left school at the end of the last term so everyone still recognised him. Several of the others stopped to talk and I heard a couple of the boys asking him what kind of job he had found.

'Oh, I'm not working yet,' he told them. 'I'm going to take a computer course.'

I had a shrewd idea that he would stick to that, just to please his parents. As he had managed to do what he did selling drugs to make money, I doubted if taking a course would stop giving that lucrative sideline.

When he looked up and saw me, a big beaming smile came onto his face. 'Hi, Amy,' he said and the sound of his voice made me smile back.

'I'm off now,' he told his friends when I reached his side. 'Coffee shop, Amy?' he asked.

'Yes, I'm dying for a big mug of it.'

As we walked away, he took my overnight bag and held my hand as we headed for our favourite coffee shop. It was once we had sat down and the steaming mugs of coffee were placed in front of us that I asked if he had brought the 'stuff' for me. 'It's been five days since I took any,' I told him. 'And I'm not feeling that good.'

'Of course I've brought it for you. I thought you might need a hit. There's a few doses in there, so be careful with it,' he told me as he passed the tiny package over to me under the table. 'You've got enough of the other stuff you need to heat it, haven't you?'

'I have,' I answered as I slid the package into my bag. I'd got quite used to injecting myself by this time as I'd been on it for a few months by now.

I didn't tell him much about what had happened between Dad and me, only about his marriage to a Thai woman.

'Is he mad? I've heard about those women out there. Many of them are prostitutes and always on the lookout for a gullible and rich man.'

'But Dad's not rich,' I protested.

'Compared to the locals out there, he is. He'll find out soon enough that it's his wallet and not his body that she's interested in. So, when's he going back there?'

'I dunno, but I think pretty soon.'

'Let's get over to Jacqui's now. I wish I could stay there with you,' he said with a charming smile which made me melt.

'But my parents wouldn't be pleased if I didn't come home. Might think I'd crashed the car.'

'Or been picked up by the police,' I said teasingly.

'Oh, they think I'm golden and I want it to stay that way.'

I had thought that Pete's solicitor was his family's but he told me that he was his own solicitor and he paid the bills directly so his parents were blissfully ignorant.

Jacqui was her usual friendly self when we arrived and told me that her daughter Sophia would sleep in with her, so I could have her bedroom. Donna was in her living room with some of her friends, who all greeted us cheerfully. As usual the stone jar got onto the table and cider was poured out for me. I glugged it down – I really would have taken anything to make me feel better.

Around eight o'clock, everyone including Pete left, which meant I was free to go upstairs. Jacqui was not someone who stayed awake long after a drinking session, and besides, she had been knocking it back all day judging by the empty wine bottles at her side.

Almost as soon as I got into the bedroom, I fumbled for everything I needed to inject myself. I can still smell it now, the aroma of the liquid that bubbled in the spoon. I almost feel that strap tied tightly round my arm to make my vein stand out. Like many addicts, I had a needle fixation which made me relax as the sting of it sent a burning feeling all the way up my arm because of the citric acid. That was when I would fall back on my pillow while every hurt feeling left my mind, leaving me happy.

I must have woken up in the early hours, feeling both

sleepy and far less miserable. Just as I tried to relax and fall back to sleep again, the picture of my dad's cold face drifted into my mind.

Got to rid myself of that, I told myself as I picked up everything needed for another hit. Again, I felt my body falling back on the pillows and that's all I can remember of the night.

If it hadn't been for Sophia, coming into her bedroom to fetch some clothes, I doubt if I would still be around to tell my story. Being really fond of me, she tried to wake me. She wanted to say good morning and to have a little chat before she left for school. When my eyes didn't open, she pinched my toes. It was then, when I didn't move, that she was scared that I was dead and screamed. That was enough to get Jacqui into the room.

After taking one look at the paraphenalia I had left beside the bed, she recognised what it was and phoned for an ambulance. She had to give the ambulance crew Dad's details as my next of kin – she was not a relative and I was underage.

I don't remember anything, not being put on a stretcher, not being carried down the stairs and nothing at all about the journey to the hospital. When I finally woke up, I had no idea where I was. As my eyes flickered around the room, I heard a voice saying, 'You're awake.' A young woman was bending over me. Looking back, I think I was a bit frightened then. I know the nurse tried to explain where I was. I remember seeing that there was a tube in my arm. She asked if I was thirsty as she tried to prop me up a little so I could drink some water.

I must have drifted back to sleep because my next memory

was being told that my father was waiting to see me. Glancing at my watch, I saw that it was just after one o'clock.

'What happened to me?' I asked the ward sister who had suddenly appeared.

'You took too much of the drugs you had with you,' she explained. 'You're lucky that someone found you so soon. Your father's here,' she added. Hardly good news, I felt – he was the last person I wanted to see.

He sat by my bed and looked down at me with an expression of distaste.

'How long have you been taking drugs?' he asked.

'A few months.'

'And where do you get them? I've been over to that house where you stayed. The woman there told me she didn't know you were taking anything until she saw the syringe by your bed.'

There was no way I was going to tell him about Pete.

'Drugs are easy to get,' was all I said. I'm sure he knew then that I must have had a dealer, but he was not about to cross-examine me there.

'The doctor here will tell you how dangerous it is to inject yourself with heroin. Because that's what it was, wasn't it, Amy?'

'Yes.'

'There's a clinic that will help you,' he told me, handing me an envelope. 'There's a couple of hundred in there and the address and telephone number of the clinic. They'll give you medicine that will help you. You're old enough to make your choice. I'm not telling Anne or your aunt about this because, if they knew, they wouldn't want you in their homes. I'll tell you something too: no one trusts a drug addict and no one wants them near them. I'm off to Thailand again tomorrow, but I'll be back in a few months. If you follow my advice, I might take you to Thailand next time. If not, be absolutely sure, I'll wash my hands of you. Do you understand me?'

'Yes.'

'So, do it right now, Amy. If not for your sake, do it for your late mother,' and with that final barb ringing in my ears, he stood up and left the room.

Maybe if he had given me a hug, looked concerned, not icy cold, his advice would have sunk in. Then I would have opened the envelope, looked at the address of the clinic and decided to do just what he had suggested. But as you will suspect, I didn't do any of those things. Instead, I put the envelope in my locker, where it stayed until I left.

It was the nurse who, seeing it, placed it in my bag.

'There's a lot of money in there. You can feel it,' she told me.

'I know.'

But I didn't open it for a long time.

24

I only need to glance down at my wrist to where the scar is to remember the day that wound on my arm occurred. A small part of how it happened was my fault but the larger part of culpability for the length and depth of the scarring lies with the police.

I'll start off with the part that was down to me. I had an accident where I fell on a piece of sharp metal that cut into my wrist. It was on a day when our teacher, Miss Simmons, had taken a group of us for a nature walk through the woods – she wanted us to learn the names of the trees and the wild flowers that grew there. I could tell she was upset when I fell on an animal trap which was hidden by the flowering gorse, especially when I yelled loudly with the sudden pain and shock of it. Miss Simmons rushed over to me, helped me up and examined the cut, which was bleeding profusely. She said that we had all better go back to the school so that my arm could be looked at by a qualified first aider then placed an arm around my shoulders to help me walk – the shock of the accident and the sight of gushing blood was making me feel quite dizzy.

It was not a huge cut but, after it was cleaned with antiseptic and bandaged, the head said that I had better go to the hospital to have it checked out: 'You might need a few stitches. It's close to a vein,' she told me. 'Don't worry, I'll take you there now.'

The thought of a needle sewing me up was enough to make me feel weak at the knees and slightly sick. I clenched my other hand tightly as my inner voice told me that I daren't faint, *It would make you appear weak if you did and you don't want to look like that, do you?*, it whispered. And no, I didn't. You might wonder why someone who injected heroin into her veins happened to be so squeamish, but somehow this was different.

I thanked the head as we got into her car and the doctor who stitched up the wound neatly, half an hour later.

'It will only be a tiny scar once it's healed,' he said reassuringly.

It would probably have ended up almost invisible by now, if a policeman hadn't managed to turn my small wound into a much larger one.

Another question you might ask is, how did the policeman do that and why?

To be honest, it was because there was an arrest warrant out for me, but I wasn't the only person to blame for that. The two officers who had brought me in with Pete a while back must have been rubbing their hands with glee when they knew that, finally, they had a good reason to arrest me.

So, what had I done? I did say I got up to mischief, didn't I? I was given a dare. It was a bet that one of the gangs of shoplifters Pete orchestrated had made with me. That was something else about him that I had previously been unaware of. It was quite a while later that I found out that he enjoyed organising others to commit the sort of petty crimes he was unwilling to be caught doing himself. If one of their number told the police it was him who told them to do it, what proof would there be? Especially as all those in the group were drug-takers. The police might have known what he was up to and hoped that he would slip up one day, but so far, he hadn't.

So, what was my dare? To prove I wasn't a stuck-up little girl, I had to pinch a few items of make-up from a department store. And yes, I got caught. Silly me, I hadn't noticed the security guard not far from where I was, watching me sneaking a few things into my bag. He waited until I was near the door and then pounced.

'I was thinking of something else, then I remembered I hadn't paid. I was just about to turn round and go to the cashier,' I said as indignantly as I could.

Clearly, he didn't believe a word I said.

'I saw you take that stuff and put it in your bag, so don't lie! You're coming with me to the manager's office,' he told me.

'Caught a thief here,' he said as he pulled me through the door. 'There's stuff in that bag of hers that's not been paid for. I caught her just as she was heading for the door.'

I should have given the manager the same excuse I had given the security man but then I didn't know much about the law. If I had, I would have made it clear that I had not actually left the store with the items and he had caught hold of me while I was still on the premises.

That guard had already snatched my bag from me and, with a smug grin, he turned it upside down on the manager's desk. There wasn't much inside – just a few lipsticks, a bottle of nail varnish and a mascara. Thank goodness I hadn't got any trace of drugs in it.

'I think we'd better phone the police, don't you, sir?'

'Well, there's not that much in that bag,' the manager said but, just as he was about to say something to me – no doubt a bit of a ticking-off – the guard butted in.

'Can't have these youngsters draining all the profits, can we? That's why I'm here, isn't it?'

That sentence was enough to make the manager phone the police.

Luckily for me it was a young constable who led me out to his car before telling me to sit in the back.

'Can't say it was a huge amount you nicked. Not that you should have done that, of course.'

I guessed then that the police would have preferred the manager to take those items off me, give me a dressing-down and threaten that, if I did it again, the police would be called. Usually that was enough to stop schoolkids from stealing again. The police would then have more time to try to stop more serious crimes.

It was Jeremy that I rang once I was at the police station. I still had his card in my bag and the young policeman allowed me to call him. He turned up fast and asked a few questions, not that there were many he could ask. He made a note that I had not left the shop when I was nabbed.

'Trouble is, that's your word against his, unless there's CCTV footage,' he told me. 'He must have been pretty new to the job not to wait until you were a few inches out the door before he grabbed hold of you,' he added with a wry smile.

'I wish I had known that then,' I said as innocently as possible. 'I would have told him again that I was just about to turn round and go to the cashier.'

'You stick to that story, Amy. You don't need to say anything else.'

A remark that told me that, although he probably knew I was guilty of shoplifting, he didn't want me to say any more in front of the police. He made it clear that he could probably get me off this time – 'But don't get up to mischief again, do you hear me, Amy? I don't want to see you being sent to a Young Offenders Detention Centre. That wouldn't be good for you.'

I was pretty nervous when I left the police station, knowing I had to appear in court. What would Anne say if she found out? Up until then she didn't know about anything about the other side of my life. She hadn't even heard about me being in hospital. Dad had managed to cover that up – he didn't want her to say that she couldn't have me staying there any longer if I might be a bad influence on her own children.

I had to think of an excuse – well, two, in fact – for the day I was due in court. One for Anne, telling her I was going to a friend, and one for the school, saying I was unwell.

Did I feel guilty that Anne trusted me? I knew that she believed I was a sensible and studious young teenager, so yes,

I did. I told her the same as I had before, that I was staying at a friend's house for a couple of nights so that we could do our homework together. She just smiled and said, 'OK, Amy, see you when you come back.' When I picked up my small overnight case as well as my satchel, I could feel my face burning with shame. She had always been so kind to me ever since my mother had been taken into hospital. I suppose I wasn't technically lying about going to a friend's house, as it was Jacqui's I was staying at, but the lie about doing homework together was blatant.

When I had asked Jacqui if I could stay there again, the answer was, 'Provided you're not going to overdose again. That little episode frightened the life out of Sophia too.'

I said I was sorry and then I had to explain about the court day – I just didn't think to tell her the time I was due to appear, which was early in the morning. I also managed to persuade her to phone the school in the morning pretending to be Anne and tell them I was unwell and needed a couple of days off.

I had tried to put on a brave face in front of Anne, but that didn't work with Jacqui. She could tell I was in a mess. If I hadn't been, I wouldn't have made the mistake of injecting myself twice in a short time. She told me that my brief stay in hospital didn't seem to have made me feel any better.

'Tell me what it is that's upsetting you so much, Amy,' she said.

Considering how much she drank, I was surprised that she had noticed and wanted me to talk about it.

'I told you Dad got married without even letting me know beforehand, didn't I? Now he doesn't want me around him.'

'But he came to the hospital, didn't he? What was it he had to say to you then?'

I explained what he had said about me taking drugs.

'He's right, you know. Alcohol's one thing and that's bad enough, but drugs are something else. The damage they do, both to the body and the head, is far worse. I think you should take his advice, don't you?'

'Isn't weed a drug?'

'Yes, but it's like comparing drinking half a pint of a lemonade shandy to downing a bottle of whisky. And even that's nothing like as dangerous as what you're putting inside yourself.'

'All right, I'm listening to you. I'll try to get off it later,' I told her as I could feel she was genuinely concerned about me.

'When?'

'I'll try to stop using after the court case,' I promised. 'I've got to get through that.'

But I didn't. I had such a sleepless night, tossing and turning. In the morning I was feeling so shaky, I knew I had to inject myself before I began the day. I'm still convinced that losing my father's love was the main reason my body had increased its need for more heroin. Looking back, I can say that I no longer cared about myself. I was definitely suffering from depression. At that time it was only heroin that took away my sadness, though even that only succeeded for a short time. Then there was Pete around me, who took a delight in my need. Unbeknown to me then, he had made sure to supply me – which meant I had to stay close to him.

He kept telling me that I mustn't miss my shot or else I

would be ill and, remembering what that was like, I went along with this advice. He was so confident that he had me under his control that he didn't mind teaching me how to inject myself with the heroin he supplied me with. He never asked for money but he also gave me small amounts so I had to keep going back to him. Not that I minded at all as unfortunately, he was the one I wanted to be with then, the one I believed I could rely on. Was it love? Of course not. I believed that the drug was my friend. Now I know it was always my enemy; an enemy that blocked me taking myself to the magistrates court, which caused a warrant to be issued for my arrest. Big mistake. So why hadn't I done what the law said and taken myself off to court?

I have to admit that the drug I took was my enemy. It should have been evident that day when I woke up after too little sleep and it was telling me I needed it badly. When my eyes opened, I felt so ill, my whole body seemed to be shaking. The only thing that would take the pain away was an injection and I believed that, if I took it, all would be well. So, I got my string out, heated the spoon with the heroin in it before shooting it into my taut arm. As the drug slid up my veins, the hit made me reel. All the tension and shakes left me, making everything around me feel so calm and peaceful. Relieved, I lay back on the bed. The problem was that, even though the drug might have removed my tension, it also took away my memory of what I was meant to be doing that day. Instead of lying there, I should have jumped out of bed, got myself dressed and readied myself to get to the court.

That was my excuse to myself then, but I now believe that

I couldn't bring myself to go to the court. Whatever the reason, it was a stupid one, wasn't it? I should have been more scared of who would be trying to find me then than how annoyed Jeremy would be.

The law then would have been that the police should have gone to the address where I was staying and explained to Anne the problem – such as the warrant with my name on it – and told her not to worry too much. As I was only thirteen, she could come with me and the solicitor would be there as well. But I know now that was not the way those policemen wanted it done – they wanted to find me somewhere on the street.

What I should have done was to get hold of Jeremy and ask for his help. I can't imagine what excuse I could have given for not turning up on time. I suppose I might have told him that I had been so sick with nerves during the evening and night that I didn't sleep until dawn. When I eventually got some sleep, it was so deep, I didn't hear my alarm go off. I realised when I woke that I had slept in, panicked about being late and couldn't face arriving late and getting into more trouble.

Whether he believed me or not, I know now that he would have done his best to sort it out, especially as I didn't have an adult to take me to court. Back then, I just felt so guilty about letting him down that I pushed the thought of getting in touch with him to the back of my mind. Also, I didn't want to tell Jacqui that I hadn't gone. Seeing as her son had served time in prison, she would have been annoyed at my stupidity. So, knowing she was still in her bedroom, I called out goodbye and scarpered.

I wasn't sure where I should go. I doubted the police had

Anne's details – I certainly never gave them to them. At least I hoped not or she would be another person I was making angry. If they visited Dad's address, they would have found it deserted.

It didn't take me long to realise that they wanted to catch me on my own and drag me back to the police station without a protective adult nearby.

It's amazing what drugs can do to the brain. I should have known full well that those bully boys who had brought Pete and me into the police station would be the ones out looking for me. They must have been over the moon when they had the reason to arrest the girl who had refused to give them the information they wanted.

It was the larger one, whose bulky frame must have been over six feet tall, who frightened me most that time. I mean, he was huge. With his cropped hair and the ugliest pair of glasses I had ever seen, it's a wonder he's not still looming about in my nightmares. With his colleague – the tall, skinny one with the bald head that the light bounced off – they were easy to spot on the street.

Those two must have been delighted when a warrant for my arrest was issued after I hadn't turned up for court. They must have hoped that I might be walking around the town. I was often at Jacqui's, so that was also a possibility. I really wasn't expecting anything to happen to me so soon after I missed my court appearance. I was on the main road going through town when I saw the bulky policeman in a car on the opposite side of the road, looking straight at me through the window. The moment I spotted him, I ran as fast as I could, but given I was on the pavement where lots of other people were walking, my progress was slowed.

The sergeant must have been really out of breath when he caught up with me. Now, what would a normal policeman have done? Perhaps just wrapped his hand around my arm and said, 'You're nicked!' as they did on TV and then waited for his partner to bring the car to where we were standing. However, that sergeant was neither normal nor ethical. Instead of doing the predictable, he flew at me with a full-on rugby tackle that sent me tumbling to the ground with him partly on top of me. I was barely seven stone then and it's a wonder he didn't do me more harm when he then kneeled and placed all his considerable weight on my back. I could hear passers-by shouting at him to get off me.

'I'll report you for this,' one man shouted. 'She's winded and you're hurting her.'

'She's a child, for God's sake!' another one yelled.

It should have bothered him much more than it appeared to as more people gathered round, pleading with him not to hurt me. Just as he shouted back that I was a criminal who had to be taken in, his colleague pulled the car over, jumped out and told people to back away.

Handcuffs were dangled in front of my face as I was pulled up. 'Don't put them on me, please,' I told him, holding out my hand, which was sporting a dressing. 'I've got stitches in my wrist.'

'Why? Did you try and kill yourself?' he sneered as he glanced at my damaged wrist. 'Anyway, too bad,' was his response as he pulled my arms round to my back, putting the cuffs on as tightly as possible. I heard a woman's voice say it wasn't legal to handcuff children.

'It is for this one!' he shouted, clicking them shut as I cried out in pain.

He had begun twisting the handcuffs so that they pulled on the stitches in my wrist.

There was no need for any of his actions because, apart from my short sprint, I hadn't tried to resist arrest – at seven stone I would hardly have been able to anyhow.

'For heaven's sake, let's get her in the car so we can get away from this group of do-gooders. Let's go!' his colleague yelled.

The officer could have just told me to get in; instead, his hand pressed the top of my head down so hard that my knees almost buckled.

'Give me your parents' name!' called out the man who had tried to defend me.

The officer in the car tried to stop me shouting back, but I managed to give the man Jeremy's name instead of Anne or Dad's as I was pushed into the back of the car. By then, the pain from the ripped stitches was excruciating and I could feel something wet soaking my sleeve.

I nearly blacked out on that short drive to the station. I felt so dizzy and sick, but I was determined not to be. Soon the car was slowing down and I knew we must be at the station when I heard the first officer's voice saying, 'Bloody hell, what's our inspector doing here?' That made me open my eyes and I saw that there was a tall grey-haired man standing just out side the doors. I could tell that the two officers were worried as the car pulled up.

It was the inspector who opened the back door and gently helped me out. I think he looked shocked when he saw the blood running down my hand.

'I want those cuffs off her straight away. Give me the key for them now.'

'She was resisting, sir, that's why they're on.'

'The key, sergeant, now!' he barked as he held his hand out. I could tell he was angry, not with me but with them, as he undid the cuffs.

To make matters worse for the two bullies, just as the cuffs came off, another car with Jeremy driving it pulled up. He stepped out of his car and walked over to where I was standing. Now those bullies looked really frightened when they saw the solicitor inspecting my bleeding arm.

'This is an attack on a minor,' Jeremy said loudly. 'Inspector, I've already got a statement about what your sergeant and his partner did to my client from a man who witnessed everything. As soon as he contacted me, I rang your station and told the duty officer to get a doctor here.'

'I know, he's already on his way,' the inspector told him. 'Now let's get inside. I think Amy needs a hot, sweet drink. And you two,' he said, turning to the bullies, 'can wait outside my office. I'll talk to you when I'm ready.'

'Yes, sir,' came the reply, which made me hope that they were shaking in their boots.

It was the inspector and Jeremy who walked in with me. I was relieved that nothing was said about me not being at the magistrates' court that day. From the way the inspector had helped me out of the car, I didn't think anything much was going to be said about that. Both of them had other things on their minds.

A hot, sweet cup of tea was brought in for me almost as soon as I sat down in the inspector's office. The doctor, who was dressed casually in jeans and a leather jacket, turned up just as I had finished it. He took hold of my arm very gently and examined it.

'I'm going to bandage it, Amy, and then you will have to be taken to the hospital. It will need some new stitches, which I can't do here,' he said.

'She needs to go now,' he told the inspector. I could tell the doctor was disgusted at the damage those handcuffs had done to what had been a minor injury, though he himself had been very gentle with me.

My wrist was so badly damaged that the doctor at the hospital told both Jeremy and I that I would have to stay in for a night. He explained to us what type of procedure would have to be done.

'We have to make sure there's no dirt left inside this wound before it's stitched,' he told me.

'Will that hurt much more?'

'No, you'll be given anaesthetic,' he told me with a comforting smile.

Now that scared me – what would happen if he saw the needle marks in my arm?

'Let's roll up your sleeve,' he told me as he gently pushed it well above my elbow. *Phew, that was lucky!* my inner voice murmured as it was my right arm without any puncture marks that he had chosen to jab the anaesthetic into.

It might not have been a serious operation, but it took quite a long time. I remember being wheeled into the theatre after my injection and feeling drowsy but I don't recall when I was wheeled back to the ward. I had been allocated a bed as soon as I was examined and awaiting the procedure. Not having anything apart from my bag, I was given a nightie that tied at the back to put on. Jeremy had left me there to go to Anne's. Knowing this would worry me, he did not tell me, but Anne did when she arrived. Yes, she was angry that I had got into trouble, but far more so about what the police bullying had done to require that I had to stay in hospital for the night.

'Whatever were you doing, Amy?' she asked in the morning when I was wide awake and not looking too bad.

'It was a stupid dare,' I told her.

'You should have told me about the court. I would have taken you there, then nothing would have happened. Jeremy has told me that you won't have to go. Thanks to him, the charges have been dropped. Now promise me you won't get up to that kind of mischief again.'

'I won't,' I told her, meaning it then.

She then told me that she would have to tell Dad what had happened. 'Don't worry too much,' she said when I looked a little scared. 'I'll tell him that you hadn't walked out of the store door, even though it's obvious that you were about to. You were, weren't you?'

'Yes,' I whispered, feeling more ashamed than ever.

'Anyhow, you won't remember it but your dad was a miner who went on strike. He's not exactlty a fan of the police in our area; he'lll never trust them, far less like them. Hearing what they did to you will bring him back. Whatever you think, you are still his daughter and he'll be furious, I promise. Now, let's get you up, Amy, and we'll go home. The ward sister has told me that you can go home now.'

Anne didn't say another word about what I'd been up to. I think she must have thought that I'd been punished more than enough for stealing a few items of make-up. What I found out a little later was that those two policemen had been forced to resign.

I never saw them again.

25

If Jeremy was furious about how the police had acted, then so, too, was my father. Anne was absolutely right in saying that neither he nor his friends had ever forgiven the police for being on Margaret Thatcher's side during the long and brutal miners' strike, the prime minister who saw it as a golden opportunity to break the unions and close the mines. Anne had also been right when she told me that she was certain that my dad would be on the phone. Not that I had believed that he would, but I was wrong there. In fact, I had been back at Anne's for less than an hour when she called out to me that Dad was on the phone and he wanted to talk to me.

'How is your arm now, Amy?' he asked immediately.

I remember thinking that it was the first kindly question that I had heard him ask in a long time.

'Not too bad, Dad, I've plenty of painkillers.'

'There's my gutsy daughter. Now when do you have to see the hospital doctor again?'

'I have an early-morning appointment in three weeks' time. The doctor told me it should have healed by then.'

'I hope so. When Anne told me what had happened, I thought that you deserved a holiday in the sun. We will have to wait and see if that's your last appointment, but then I think a few weeks away would help you recover. Do you agree?'

'Do you mean you want me to come to Thailand, Dad?'

'Of course. I know it's a place you're going to love and the Thai food here's so much better than what we get in the UK. And no, you won't have to travel over here on your own. I need to come back to England for a while – I've some business to sort out, so you and I can go on the plane together.'

There was a pause. He knew that I would have understood that his wife would be with us on the holiday he was offering me. I might not have been happy at that, but I wanted to see my father. I really had thought that we were unlikely to ever be friendly again and, despite how much he had upset me, I couldn't help missing him.

I surprised myself when I felt a surge of joy at his offer. He was actually sounding a bit like the old dad, the one I had missed ever since Mum left us. Once I said that I would love to go to Thailand with him, he changed the subject to what he thought about the police and their brutality. He cursed 'those wretched men in blue' as he called them for what they had done to me. Even over the phone I could hear the anger he felt. I almost thought that the hatred I could hear in his voice when he said, 'How dare they injure my young daughter,' was even greater than his concern for me. Still, when he finally got off that subject and asked me the question that I had dreaded hearing, he actually sounded warm and friendly towards me. It was that approach which compelled me to give him a truthful answer.

'Have you opened the envelope I left you with in the hospital?'

'No, not yet, Dad,' I answered, waiting for him to tick me off.

To my surprise he sounded a little amused when he said, 'Well then, I suppose you've not contacted the clinic yet either? Now this is what you've got to do when this call ends. Get that envelope open, there's money in it to pay for medical help. That is, if you seriously want this holiday. Apart from the money, there's a note inside with all the details of the clinic, the address and the phone number. I spoke to them before I left the UK so they have your name written down, which means they'll see you. Now listen to me, Amy, I want you to understand that you have to be careful because very few doctors will give people of your age the prescriptions that you will need.'

'You mean they're not supposed to, don't you?'

'Yes, but they put the needs of young addicts in front of their careers. They're remarkable people. It's the only place where you can get help. You mustn't tell anyone about it either, which I explain in the note I left for you. I know I can trust you there.'

'You can, Dad,' I said sincerely.

'There's a doctor there who will give you the prescription for methadone.' He then went on to tell me what happens to anyone young or old who tries to smuggle illegal drugs into Thailand. Boy, that got through to me. I had heard how some drug smugglers had been caught and how they had disappeared into prison system for years. Being there without the ability to inject myself was a little worrying but I was determined then to do my best to come off the drug I had been on, if that meant I could travel abroad to be with my father.

When the call was finished, I did as he had asked and took the envelope out of the drawer where I had placed it. I read his notes and then made the phone call.

The next morning, still being signed off from school, I told Anne that I was off to the shops to get a few things with the money Dad had left for me. Without asking what it was I wanted, she just smiled and said, 'OK, love, see you later.'

I wondered if she would have used the term 'love' had she known what I was going out for. Head down, I went straight to the address my father had given me.

I'm not including the name of the clinic or describing where it was, or anything else about it here in this book because of what Dad had explained to me. The people at the clinic understood that there were dealers who made money in getting youngsters onto their list of customers. They had decided it was their duty to help all ages of vulnerable people to get off drugs before the addiction destroyed their young lives.

I was seen immediately and, after answering some questions about my personal background and medical history, we got onto my heroin intake. Almost straight away, I received my prescription for methadone and was given helpful instructions by the doctor in how to use it because the medicine was in tablet form – 'It will help you make you relax, but for a while it will also make you a little sleepy,' he told me.

I suppose because of my age, he asked a lot of questions around how long I had been taking heroin.

'Since I was twelve,' I told him. There was something about that doctor that made me tell him how I had started and how I had been led to believe that just one injection had made me an addict. I described how ill I had felt after the first one. 'It was the second that made me feel better,' I told him.

'Is it from that person that you still get your heroin?'

'Yes, he doesn't let me pay anything for it either.'

I could see him frowning then and I knew there were more questions that he wanted the answer to.

'You said "he", so is the person you are talking about your boyfriend?'

'Not really,' I said because I hadn't seen Pete as that for quite a while. It was when I came to know about him organising youngsters to shoplift that I began to use excuses not to see him. Now if the methadone helped me enough to give up the heroin, I wouldn't have to either.

The doctor didn't ask anything more then and changed the subject to my holiday.

'Your dad has told me about taking you to Thailand once your wrist is healed. You know that you cannot have any heroin in your blood when you go, don't you?'

'Yes, Dad told me that.'

Actually, I know now that blood tests were unlikely to be given at the airport but then the doctor was aware that there were people who mixed heroin with methadone. He wanted to make sure that I wasn't temped to do that.

He continued to reinforce what Dad had already warned

me about. That anyone who got caught with drugs on them in Thailand would look forward to being in a very terrible prison for a very long time – 'That's why your dad wants me to make sure you have the medicine you need when you go.'

I thanked him then for I was feeling grateful, though I had the feeling when I left that there was more – apart from him wanting to know the date I was leaving – that he wanted to discuss with me.

My next stop was the chemist that the doctor had told me to go to. I handed over the prescription and received my first packet of methadone. Once I got back to Anne's, I went up to my room and took my first tablet. It was nothing like the drug I had been taking for nearly two years. I didn't feel it running up my arteries, nor did I fall back on my pillows as I was taken into the world of ecstasy it created.

With this obvious difference between the two drugs, how did I like methadone? Well, not as much as heroin, but the word 'freedom' was what I hung onto. For didn't I want a life without drugs? A life where it was safe to travel. A life where I didn't have to lie about being an addict. Because that, I told myself, was what I was. It was those thoughts that made me see the benefit of my new prescription. Apart from being able to swallow and not inject into my veins, they made me relax and it took away the depression which failed to leave me and replaced it with a wave of happiness.

* * *

At my hospital appointment three weeks later, the doctor examined my arm, took out the stitches and told me I was free to go to Thailand. When I looked down at the undressed wound, I felt sick. That scar was so red and raw.

'That redness will fade a lot over the next few months. Just don't try and hide it with a bracelet. You mustn't have anything rubbing on it and keep it out of the sun,' I was told. The doctor gave me a prescription of a certain type of cream that I could rub it very gently with.

'Long sleeves for me then,' I said, trying to grin.

'You enjoy your holiday, Amy,' was all he said, giving me a friendly pat on the shoulder.

Since the phone call from Dad inviting me there, I was really looking forward to going to Thailand. I had been wondering how I could as there were no long school holidays due. Still, that was for Dad to sort out, so I did as I had been asked and sent him a message telling him that the doctor had told me my arm had healed well and I could now travel.

He rang a few hours later to tell me that he was booking to come home and then, about a week later, we would be flying to Thailand together.

'But what about school?' I asked.

'You think you might be suspended for playing truant if you come with me?' he said, laughing a little. 'Don't worry, I've already spoken to the head. I told him what you've been through and he's agreed to you having some time off. You must bring some homework with you, but not too much as the school wants you to have a good time.'

I still don't know how my father managed it. My guess now

is that he used the fact that I hadn't met his new wife – my stepmother – yet. Meeting her would have sounded important. I'm sure he must have told the head that he was bringing his wife to England once her visa was sorted out. That might have made the head feel that it was important that some kind of relationship needed to be established between us before she arrived in the UK. I was never told how Dad managed to arrange for me to go back with him to Thailand, but I'm pretty sure that I got the story right.

As soon as Dad sent me the message with the dates of my trip, I made my appointment at the clinic to obtain the prescription I would need. I also made sure my teachers had the dates of my holiday so that they could get my study tasks ready.

The following day, I went along to my appointment at the clinic as soon as school came out. The doctor noted down the dates and told me that he would give me a prescription to cover that time.

'How's the methadone working for you, Amy?'

'I'm managing with it,' I told him.

'Good for you. Now listen to what I'm telling you. The prescription you're getting is for the whole time you're going to be there. You mustn't open the packages. You have a separate one to carry you through until you go and for the two weeks after you return. Leave it at home when you depart. The one you're taking with you will be sealed with the prescription on it – the script on it makes the package appear safe. Your dad's going to carry it in his hand luggage.

'You take your last tablet on the day of your flight. Do not carry even one tablet with you in your luggage.'

'Why?'

'Sniffer dogs are used in the airports, that's why.'

'Right, I've got the message,' I told him.

That doctor was one courageous man. He was dedicated to helping those who needed him. I learnt a long time later that he left the UK to join the group of medical people called Doctors Without Borders. They risk their lives when they fly into poverty-stricken and war-torn zones to help the sick and the wounded.

He certainly did his best to help me. Not once, but twice.

26

In the end it's hope that destroys us, not despair.
That I know only too well.
I believed it was love that had taken me to Thailand.
It was, but not for the love of me.

I wrote that on the cover of a notebook when I returned from Thailand. Inside were some photos of myself and Chelsea, a friend I made while I was there. There were some of me dancing and others when I was in a big group of young Thai people. Also, a newspaper clipping with my photo on it – I'll explain exactly how that got there later! As I flicked through the pages and read my notes, I remembered exactly what my time there had been like and just about everything that I got up to on that holiday.

People often say it, and travel brochures reiterate repeatedly, that Thailand is a land of smiles. Not for me, it wasn't. Within a couple of days, I knew that my dad and I would never bond together ever again. I can rationalise it now, but

I didn't understand it then – no matter what has gone wrong, children keep hoping that their parents will show them that they're loved. They will try to gain happy smiles, hugs and reassuring words from them, but if they don't succeed, then there's no anchor to keep their feet firmly on the ground. Children need stability in their lives, especially after their equilibrium has been unbalanced by trauma.

Just meeting Dad's new wife made it clear that what I had believed after that first phone call from him was the truth. The friendly, more recent calls were mainly to persuade me to do what he wanted.

I had jumped at the invitation to visit Thailand because I wanted to be as close to Dad as I had been before Mum died. However much I kept telling myself not to care, underneath, I was miserable about us not being on speaking terms. I still wasn't looking forward to meeting the woman he had married, but I knew this was something I had to do. I might have hoped, when we were talking on the phone, that we were getting closer, but Dad still made it clear that he expected me to be pleasant to his wife when we met and to welcome her to our family. He might not have spelt it out this time, but I had a feeling that if I wasn't, he would go back to being that unloving father who had made me cry so often. The question that stayed in the back of my mind was, did I want to be the daughter who was no longer important in her father's life?

Since Dad had been going out to Thailand, I had heard a lot of rumours about why single men went there on holiday and not very nice ones too. I had also listened to my aunts and

Anne talking when I was not in the room, saying it was lonely men the women there wanted to ensnare so that they could get their hands on their money. After that, I had no reason to believe otherwise. In fact, I had every reason to believe every single word I had heard was true.

If I had a reason not to want to think of her as my new mother or even my stepmother, for me, that was one of the main issues. It was bad enough accepting the fact that he had married her, but suspecting she was fleecing him did nothing to enamour me. Now I can see that, in my father's mind, his offer to take me to Thailand was so that I could meet her. Even all these years later, I can never understand how he believed that any new wife would be a replacement mother for me. He had seen how long it had taken me to get over Mum's death. Surely, he should have realised why I could never bring myself to call another woman 'Mum'.

If he had wanted to marry again, maybe I could have accepted that but wasn't I old enough to call her by her first name? That I could have handled, but not the name I called my mother. The thought of her walking through our front door and me having to call out, 'Hello, Mum,' was enough to make me shudder.

* * *

I didn't go back to the house when Dad arrived. He had told me he had a lot to do while he was there, not that I knew then what it was. It would be better for me if I stayed at Anne's, he said.

'Don't want you being there on your own. I expect you'll need to pack some summer things, so here are the keys so you can let yourself in,' he told me as he placed them in my hand. 'Now, how much of the two hundred I left you do you still have?'

'Most of it.'

'Good for you! Seeing as you've been careful with it, here's another hundred. You'll need a couple of summer dresses for Thailand. Take yourself off to the shops to get anything you need. Don't forget to buy some sun cream to take with you. Mind you get a high factor, it's extremely hot and humid there. But shopping there is also great – you can even get things made up for you in a matter of days. You've got your prescription sorted, haven't you?'

'Yes, Dad, and thanks for the cash.'

'Good! How are your new meds working for you?'

'All right. Except they make me a bit drowsy.'

'It's bound to be different, but you haven't mixed it with any heroin, have you?'

'No, Dad, I haven't.'

'I believe you – you're looking better already,' he said as a warm smile came in my direction.

* * *

It was certainly a very different smile to the one on Pete's face when I told him that I was no longer going to take his drugs.

'Because you can't take them into Thailand on holiday?'

'No, because I want to be normal.'

'Mmm, do you? Wait till you come back and let's see if you don't ask for them again then.'

That was when I began to feel uneasy around him. His remark told me that he didn't want me to get clean. I should have been aware of that earlier. How I wish that I had taken note of these comments more. That might have made me wake up to his reason for giving me my first injection. I know now that it was so that he could control my younger self. Like any other dealer, he knew that addicts could never walk away from those who supplied them.

Unfortunately, my mind was not on Pete that day, it was on my needing to sort out what I wanted to take with me on holiday. Using the keys Dad had handed to me, I let myself into the house. I went straight to my bedroom so that I could sort out some summer clothes for my holiday. How I hated the feeling of emptiness that hit me the minute I walked through the door. There was no longer the warmth of people living there – it made me want to leave as quickly as I could.

On the Saturday, I took myself to Nuneaton to do the shopping Dad had suggested I might do. I found the boutique where he took me on my birthday. It was full of tempting tops, but I stuck to just buying a couple of sun dresses. Then I went to the chemist and bought plenty of factor-30 sun cream and a few other toiletries in small travel sizes. Everything else that I put in my suitcase came from my old bedroom – I was quite pleased with myself for not being tempted to buy more things and blow all the money. While on the high street, I popped into a travel agent and asked for brochures on Thailand. That night, I flipped through the pages, seeing happy tourists visiting exotic temples and palaces, night markets, enjoying elephant rides and floating markets. There were curious monkeys and visits to silk factories and places where beautiful umbrellas were hand painted. Azure beaches, exotic islands and stunning scenery. The food, the tropical fruits and exotic cocktails, all looked so enticing. As I took it all in, I could hardly wait for the holiday to begin.

27

Dad collected me from Anne's the day we were flying out to Thailand. Checking in was as easy as it had been the last time I had been on a plane. Neither of us had much to say on that flight as he told me to try and get some sleep as soon as possible after the meal because Thailand was many hours ahead of us. 'It's about early morning their time when we land, so we will have lost quite a few hours. I'm used to it, but you might struggle with jet lag. Also, the flight itself is long,' he explained.

Once our food was delivered and we had finished eating, I spent the rest of those interminable hours watching movies, listening to music and reading. I tried to sleep and managed to doze off intermittently. Dad woke me as the plane's internal lights went on, signalling that we were about to be fed again. A quick snack, a scrabble for the bathrooms and then we were getting ready to land.

'Have a look out of your window, Amy,' my father said.

As I had the window seat, I pulled up the miniature blind

to see dazzling sunlight bouncing off the glass on the airport buildings as we started to land.

Good thing I brought all that sun cream…

As soon as we were able to leave our seats, I could tell from the expression on Dad's face that he, like the other passengers, could hardly wait to get off the plane. He took down our hand luggage and, in no time at all, we were outside on the tarmac and into the scorching heat. By the time our passports were stamped and handed back to us, I was both hot and tired. On top of my lack of sleep, I wasn't completely over coming off heroin. The doctor had been right, methadone was still making me feel sleepy. I had taken a dose before we left for the airport but, having not been able to swallow another for so long, I was already beginning to feel pretty shaky. I knew where the packet containing them was: in Dad's hand luggage. They were still sealed with the script attached, which, if they saw it, would tell customs it was prescribed medicine. I couldn't blame my father for insisting that it was him, not me, who was going to carry it.

It felt like it all took a long time for us to clear customs and get out of the airport. I noticed that Dad was looking around, no doubt hoping that his Thai bride would have come to meet us. I could tell that he was disappointed that she hadn't. All I wanted to do was to get somewhere I could get some water and swallow one of my tablets. To be fair to Dad that day, he realised that and walked us over to a small café in the arrivals area – 'There's a toilet just round the corner. Take my travel bag with you and put your meds in your handbag. I've worked out that you need to take one now because of the time difference. Here's a bottle of water and I'll order you a hot drink for when you come out then we'll collect my car and head straight for our hotel.'

It might have been sweltering hot there and you might think that both of us would have wanted cool drinks, but unfortunately for me, it was the hot ones that made the methadone work faster.

Into the loo I went, swallowed what I needed, splashed cold water onto my face, combed my hair and then, already feeling better, I walked out to where Dad was sitting with his phone in his hand.

'Have that drink I've got for you,' he told me. 'Then we can go over to where my car is parked and in a couple of hours we'll be at the hotel. Dang says she will meet us there.'

Try and look as though you're looking forward to seeing her, I told myself, even though I would have liked to spend some more time with Dad on his own. What I didn't know was that it was only to be that journey where I would have Dad all to myself.

We chatted a little on the drive and, as we neared the hotel, he pointed to a wooden building with chairs and tables outside, telling me that it was a friend's bar. That hardly surprised me as it was only a few metres from the hotel where he and Dang were living. I noticed the large group of sun-tanned people sitting outside with beers and then we pulled up in front of our hotel.

I must admit that it was as breathtakingly beautiful as the one I had liked so much in Turkey. A four-star heaven, I called it, after just a couple of nights of being there.

'I'll come up to your room in about an hour or so,' my father said as we got into the lift. 'So, get yourself unpacked, have a shower and change into some lighter clothes. We'll have an early lunch and then you can nap but don't go fast asleep or you'll stay jet lagged.'

The lift stopped on the first floor for Dad to go to his room, or rather his and wife's room, and then it went up two more floors to mine. I was relieved that my room was nowhere near theirs. Even better, when the porter carried my case in, I could see it was on the opposite side of the corridor to Dad's. That meant, when I wanted to sit peacefully on my small balcony, I wouldn't find myself looking down onto theirs.

Let's get unpacked, I told myself, making sure that the first thing I did was to place my methadone in the safety deposit box in the wardrobe. It was not something I wanted the cleaners to find – that might have caused trouble if they recognised what it was. Once my tablets were in a safe place, I took off the clothes I had travelled in and then, just wearing my underwear, I opened my case and pulled out what I was going to change into after I had showered. What I really wanted to do was to lie down on that bed and sleep, but I could do that after lunch, I decided. It would be a bit rude not to eat with them on the first day I arrived.

I began hanging up my clothes and was in the middle of it when I heard knocking on the door. *If that's Dad, he's not waited for an hour*, I thought. I could hardly open the door in my underpants, could I? I called out to wait a minute as I had several garments dangling on my arm.

'Oh, just open it, Amy, we don't want to stand in this corridor much longer,' I heard him call out.

That irritated me. Why couldn't he say he would see me downstairs? Still not wanting to annoy him after we had only just arrived, I dropped everything on the floor, quickly pulled a top over my head and opened the door.

There he was, still sporting some a tan from his visit there a few weeks earlier, wearing baggy shorts and a yellow T-shirt. Standing next to him was a small dark-haired woman, forcing what I saw was an insincere smile at me.

Now what would have been the tactful introduction? Certainly not the one he gave, which was, 'Amy, this is Dang, your new mum.' I should think that anyone else would understand how I felt, especially as I was shocked at seeing the ring on her hand that had been taken off Mum's finger when she died – Dad must have taken it for Dang.

Dad had always told me that Mum's jewellery, including that engagement ring, would be mine when I was a little older. Ever since then, I had thought of how I would treasure it. I used to creep into the bedroom where once my two parents had slept together and slip that particular ring onto my wedding ring finger – it made me feel closer to Mum. Then one day it had vanished and I was worried that somehow it had been lost or stolen. I never said anything to Dad in case he blamed me for its disappearance. It was not until I saw them both at the door that I realised who had taken it and why.

Seeing that ring on a stranger's hand was like a stab to the heart. It really was the final straw. It symbolised my last tangible memory of my mother and I had fantasised about it one day being the ring I would wear a daily basis and remember her every time I saw it on my finger. I nearly burst into tears, but instead, my anger took over, putting a stop to that.

I think now that my younger self, who was so upset about the ring, might have managed to swallow her anger if Dad hadn't used the phrase 'your new mum' to introduce her. I can remember very clearly how I had more than once tried to explain to Dad why I couldn't call another person 'Mum'. That was my name for her, my own mum. Would he have liked to have a wife with the same name as the previous one? I doubt it somehow. He would have surely thought of some kind of nickname for her to use instead. Dad had obviously ignored my explanation – stubborn is barely a strong enough word to describe him.

Those words – 'your new mum' – made me shake with fury and, before I could I tell myself not to, I heard the words, 'Like fuck she is!' come flying out of my mouth.

Dad's face was like thunder. If I could be with him now, I would say, 'What did you expect? You were trying to force me to accept a new mother, which was not the same as you taking a new wife.'

Realising that I had put my foot in it, I took a deep breath – I didn't want my dad not talking to me while I was on holiday there.

'Sorry if I snapped,' I managed to say. 'I'm tired, so let me get unpacked and have that shower and rest for a bit.'

From the glare that came in my direction, I knew that excuse was not working well. Not only that, I thought by the expression on his face that he wished he hadn't brought me back with him. A question flew into my head then: why had he brought me there? There had to be a reason.

And there was. A reason I would find out soon.

I noticed Dang meeting his gaze, which made his thunderous expression change a little. All he said then was, 'All right, Amy. We'll leave you alone,' and taking hold of Dang's arm, they walked away.

For the first time since I had begun taking methadone, all I wanted was to get smashed. I wished I had been able to bring what I had thought of as my best friend with me. Just one stab in my arm would chase away those unhappy feelings that were coming fast and furiously into my mind. It would stop the tears that were threatening to slide down my cheeks straight away. I can picture myself now standing by the door, longing to feel that familiar scratch of the needle going in my arm, and then there would be the burning sensation before the hit made me forgot everything that was saddening me.

At least I had some guts left as I took notice of my inner voice telling me to be grateful, I had methadone.

Just bringing those tablets with you will rid you of your addiction. Don't think about it, heroin is NOT your friend, my inner voice told me. *Take the methadone and be grateful that you will be able to live a normal life soon.*

Yes, but there's none of the buzz that I want. And I need it now.

No, but it makes you feel better.

All right, I'll be sensible and stick to the methadone, I told myself. *After all, in a few months, I won't have to take any meds. Now I'm going to finish my unpacking.*

Then after your shower, make yourself look decent and try and get Dad friendly again, said that niggling little inner voice of mine.

That means I also have to try and be nice to Dang.

Yes. You need to try, Amy.

Come on, I told myself, *I'm going to have a nice holiday and I can go shopping. Thailand sells the most beautiful silk scarves and clothes.*

I knew that because of all my reading up. It meant that I could get a special present for Anne as well as something for myself.

Good, said the voice. *Anyhow, he'll give you more money just so you can disappear for a while.*

I realised then that was why, in the past, Dad had been so generous with it.

28

I decided to obey that inner voice of mine. I had a quick shower then, resisting the temptation to crawl back into bed, I slid into a sleeveless cream dress, gave my hair a brush, practised putting on a friendly smile in the mirror and setting my shoulders back. Then I went down to Dad's room and knocked politely on his door.

I hope he doesn't tell me to piss off, I thought to myself.

He didn't. Instead, he called out, 'Is that you, Amy?'

'Yes.'

He opened the door and very quietly told me to apologise to Dang: 'Do that, please, and then the three of us can go and get something to eat.'

Now I know that it was Dang who had encouraged him to be a little kinder. I gave her more or less the same remarks I had made earlier by way of apology: that I had been tired after the flight, though I did manage to get the word 'sorry' out.

'I understand, Amy, it's difficult for you. I don't want to take away what you felt for your mother,' she said.

I don't think for one minute that either of them believed I was being sincere, but between walking away from my room and me knocking on their door, they must have made up their minds not to row with me.

'Let's go downstairs to the hotel restaurant, the food there is good,' said Dad.

The restaurant was so nice that I was pleased I had made myself look smart. The menu had both European food as well as Thai on offer. I don't know why I chose something so ordinary, but I did. Scrambled eggs and ham and toast of all things! Perhaps it was comforting. How funny that I can still remember that.

Once the meal was finished, Dad mentioned that I most probably wanted to rest a bit and maybe sit in the sun, where I could get a tan: 'Hope you've brought your swimsuit and your sun cream with you? Don't forget how burnt you got in Turkey, so take it easy.'

'I have, and I will, Dad – I don't want to get burnt like that again.'

'Good sunbathing here needs to be done gradually,' he told me. 'Later, we can all go to Rob's Bar. He's got some good live music on tonight, I'm sure you'll enjoy that.'

That brightened me up a little, even though I got the message that they wanted to be on their own until then.

I could have gone to the pool, but instead, finding the chair on my balcony could be turned into a comfortable lounger, I decide to do my sunbathing there. I didn't really want to go outside and sit on my own amongst a group of strangers so soon. I dozed a little out there and, by the end of the afternoon, my face, arms and legs had turned a pale pink.

That pink will soon turn brown, I told myself.

At six I had another shower, which helped me cool down a little, rubbed aftersun on, then sorted out what I thought was a suitable dress for the evening: a blue one this time. On went a small amount of make-up before I brushed my hair again and then took myself down to Dad's room.

It was the live music that had encouraged me to tell myself that the evening would not be so bad. After all, what teenager who is not allowed to drink anything alcoholic in front of their father is going to enjoy watching the adults knocking back their drinks? Very few I know, anyway, seeing that nearly twenty years later, I have a teenage daughter of my own.

Both Dang and Dad looked as though they were ready when I came down to their room.

'There'll be food at the bar,' Dad told me. 'Hot dogs, burgers, that kind of thing.'

Dang and I might have taken the effort to look our best, but Dad didn't look all that different to how he had earlier. Dang, however, looked good. She was wearing a sparkling pale turquoise dress and some more jewellery, most of which I recognised as having been Mum's.

Just ignore it, I told myself, *it wasn't her who took it.*

Even before I arrived in Thailand, I had a suspicion that Dad had done that. When I had the keys to the house, I had searched everywhere to see what of Mum's jewellery was still in the room. All of it was gone; there was not one item remaining of all the pieces Mum had collected over the years. Some of them, she had told me, were presents from her family and others, apart from her engagement ring, she had bought herself. So, I had already known that Dad had removed everything and there was nothing of Mum's left. Things my parents had both promised to me. Seeing Mum's favourite necklace around Dang's neck, as well as all her rings on Dang's fingers, was hard. I was more disappointed than angry – that would come later.

'You look very nice, Amy,' said Dad.

'She does,' agreed Dang.

Somehow I managed to swallow the feelings I had – they could wait until I left Thailand.

'Lovely dress, Dang,' I managed to get out and hoped I wasn't going to be jumped on for using her name instead of the word Dad wanted to hear. But nothing was said and smiles were exchanged.

'Let's go,' said Dad and off we went to Rob's Bar.

I could hear the music as we walked over the road and towards the place. *Must be a British group,* I thought, *judging by the sound of the male singer's voice.* Once we were in, I could see that the tall blond man whose voice I liked was the only one in the group who was not Thai.

The place was already crowded and I noticed to my relief that there were quite a few younger people already on the small dance floor, swaying away to the music. None of them were quite as young as me, though, but then it was hardly the right place for someone of my age to spend the evening in – that's my dad for you.

There were a couple of girls only about three years older than me, who were dancing together. What I learnt about them later was that they often came to Rob's and they were looking for foreign men who would pay them to go to a hotel with them. Not that that would have bothered me then or now – we all have to make a living.

Seeing I was with two adults who were hardly paying me much attention, they came over to where I was sitting. Laughing away, they said, 'Come and dance,' as one of them took hold of my arm. Their English was not too bad and they were good at showing me how to move on the dance floor to the rhythm of the music.

I found myself laughing with them as I swayed and twisted my body. Feeling thirsty, when the musicians had a short break, I trotted back to the bar where Dad and Dang were perched on stools. A glass of cola came my way as at the same time they topped up their glasses with white wine. I wished I could have some, or even a nice strong glass of cider.

Before the music started up again, another young Thai woman appeared. She came over to where we were sitting and, on seeing her, Dang smiled broadly and then introduced her to Dad and me.

'Amy, this is Chelsea, a good friend of mine.'

Seeing me looking rather puzzled at the name, both women laughed. 'I'm a massive fan of Chelsea Football Club,' the newcomer told me in fluent English. 'That's why people call me that. I went to see them play as much as I could when I was at uni over there.'

It didn't take long for me to realise that Dang had a reason for inviting Chelsea over. Even though there was quite a large age gap, she thought that we would get on well. Which we did. After all, Chelsea was quite a bit younger than Dang and they appeared to be close friends. I know now that Dang had invited her so that I could have a decent holiday. She must have talked it over with Dad. Not that he needed any persuasion for me to have a friend over there who would keep me occupied and out of their way.

That evening, Chelsea certainly let me know that she was going to do her best to make my holiday a fun one. 'I think you're old enough to see some of the other clubs here, they're pretty wild,' she told me.

'That sounds a great idea,' I said, trying to stop myself from yawning, for my body clock was telling me I should have been asleep ages ago.

'Thought you'd be a party girl,' she said with a grin.

Despite our age gap, I began to feel we were two of a kind.

'There's a party I can take her to the day after tomorrow. She should have got over jet lag by then,' she said, looking at Dad.

'As long as she's not out all night,' was the answer. He didn't even ask where the party was. I suppose, as Chelsea was a friend of his wife, he trusted her to look after me.

Like my first day in Thailand, the following day, apart from joining Dad and Dang for lunch, I spent most of it on my own. I didn't want to be yawning again the next day when I was going to a party so I decided to have supper in my room and rest to get over my jet lag.

I was right, I felt so much better when I woke up in the

morning. And this time I had something to look forward to. There was also more time sunbathing and I could see I was already turning a nice shade of brown. I went down to the pool, where groups of people were enjoying the sun, and swam for about an hour before having lunch with Dang and Dad again. This time I was guided by Dang and experienced my first Thai food in Thailand. It was fantastic, but very hot.

*   *   *

That first evening out with Chelsea was great fun. She had taken me to a local club named Hollywood, where there was not one tourist apart from me and no one seemed remotely bothered at how old I was. The whole place was painted a rich, dark blue. Above our heads were glowing lights inside bamboo lampshades. Underneath my feet, the flooring was a shiny black. And at the sides of the room were high, round wooden tables with tall stools. As soon as I walked in, I found myself simply loving the colours and the sounds of the music throbbing out.

I was told that the club had large parties several times a week and that Chelsea, who had a pass for the VIP section, attended many of them. Nothing was going to stop either of us saying yes when we were told about the next party we were invited to.

I discovered that, although Thai boys had seen British girls from a distance, they had not met many of them. They certainly paid me a lot of attention as I was the only non-Thai person there. At the age I was then, I just about preened with pleasure at all the compliments coming my way and spent nearly all my time on the dance floor.

My dad didn't seem bothered at all, despite what he knew had been going on with me back in the UK. He certainly didn't seem concerned about my doing anything illegal in Thailand. Given his behaviour the whole trip, I think I was just immune to him at that time so I didn't see it. Going around with Chelsea simply made me love Thailand all the more. Now, as a mother of a teenage girl, I would not have been happy at her being out there in the early hours. There are places which are far from safe. Although I was nearly always with Chelsea, even so, it was not always a safe country, especially for young people.

29

It must have been when I was near to leaving that I found out why Dad had brought me over to Thailand. He believed that Dang was struggling to get a visa but, if she was able to show that she had just become a stepmother, then there would be far less of a problem. It was Chelsea who explained everything to me.

'There are some women who have married Western men so that they can leave Thailand. Then there have been some gay men from Europe who have paid a Thai girl to marry them so that they can stay here, where there is a big gay club scene. There's all kind of reasons for these sorts of marriages and the embassies are aware of them all. But neither of them is that young and your dad is spending a lot of time with her – it hardly looks like one of those relationships.'

'So why is Dang having all those problems? Is it because she wants to stay here?' I asked curiously.

'Think you've guessed the reason, Amy. I don't think she wants to live in England.'

'Why does Dad not realise it?'

'She says England is a cold, wet and bleak country. She wants your dad to spend most of his time over here. She understands that you'll never see her as a mother and she thinks it would be easier for you not to have her living in the house where you were born, sleeping in the bed your mother slept in. Be better if just came over here for your holidays. Wouldn't you prefer that?'

'Yes,' I answered, feeling a wave of sadness. I doubted if I would see much of Dad once I went back to the UK.

'Are you telling me this because Dang asked you to, Chelsea?'

'Let's say she dropped a hint. She's a bit concerned about you believing that her visa's taking a long time. Your dad thought that showing your passport and telling them she was your stepmother would persuade the authorities to get her visa through a lot more quickly. He even brought your birth certificate with him so that Dang can prove you are the daughter of the man she has married.'

'Dad will know what she's been up to eventually, won't he?'

'I expect so. What she's hoping is that he, like her, won't want to leave. She's already secretly looking for a house they can move into. No matter how rich he is, living in a hotel is not a long-term thing. Dang wants a proper home with him, in Thailand.'

'But Dad's not rich! Doesn't he need to work?'

I got a sympathetic look then.

'Didn't you know that he has another house? That's the one that gives him income as it's rented out.'

'No!' was my answer as my heart gave another lurch, for I had no idea about it. 'Where is that house?'

'I don't know exactly, but it's not very far from the one he lives in. From what Dang told me, he bought it before he married your mother. Maybe he was living there when he met her.'

That information made me feel even worse. It meant he hadn't needed to take Mum's jewellery, that I know she would have wanted me to have, he could just have bought Dang some new things instead. I wished I didn't, but I believed every word Chelsea said.

It was that evening that my photo with Chelsea was taken; the one that my younger self placed in her diary.

'Shall I walk you over to the hotel?' Chelsea asked, after we had finished our drinks.

For the first time since I had met her, I felt I needed some time on my own. I suppose I should have been grateful that I knew the truth. I wanted to try and digest everything that she had told me; I needed to think of what I would do once I was back in England. With all the noise in the bar, I wanted to clear my head. I thought it would be a good idea to take myself outside and sit on one of the tables there.

'No, I'm fine,' I told her. 'The hotel's only a couple of hundred yards and a quick walk might help me get my head straight.'

'Are you sure?'

But when she left, instead of going straight home, I went straight to the bar and ordered another drink: a glass of chilled white wine.

Rob's eyebrows shot up a little because he knew what age I was. 'Don't you drink too much, Amy, or your dad will be down on me,' he warned before disappearing into the back of the bar.

His words made the barman smile at me: 'Make that your last one, or I'll be in trouble,' he gently told me.

I took my glass of wine outside and sat at a table, gazing up at the stars. My mind was all over the place then. If Dad stayed here, where would I live? If I had been a little older, I could have lived in Dad's house on my own, but I would hardly want to. I suppose, while he was sending both Anne and me money, it would be her house I would stay in.

Don't give Dad any clues about what you know, I told myself. I knew it was going to be hard for me to keep a smile on my face, but I didn't want him being angry again.

So, did he want me out of his life? Though I believed then that he would do the honourable thing of making sure I was all right, I still had to accept his lack of affection for me and keep him on side.

Dang had got Chelsea to entertain me and, thinking over my excitement at looking at all the things Thailand offered, I realised I had done none of them: no markets, no elephants, no scenic boat rides. Most of the time had been spent in the hotel or the clubs and bars. Even my gift shopping had been done in the hotel shop.

When I look at that old diary of mine, it's that last photo that the barman took of Chelsea and me that evening that brings back a memory, one I really wish I didn't have. I should have let her walk me back to the hotel but then she didn't know I was going to stay on at the bar and, if she had, she would have insisted. The photo shows my younger self with my long dark hair falling on my shoulders, dressed in hot pants and a bikini top. That was an outfit that had got me a lot of attention when I walked around with Chelsea. It never entered my head that it was not a good idea to dress like that when I was on my own. I had never given any thought to personal safety until that last night out – Thailand was not always a safe place. I hadn't heard the word 'paedophile' then and, even if I had, I wouldn't have known the meaning of it.

I think Rob must have thought that I had gone back to the hotel when I left the bar, otherwise he would have come out to make sure I was safe. He had been in Thailand long enough to know that a scantily dressed young girl sitting alone outside a bar in the dark could get into serious trouble. At first I found being there in the moonlight, sipping my drink, peaceful – but it was a peacefulness that didn't last for long.

Lost in thought, my attention was seized by some untoward movement. A man was almost hidden by the shadows. As I watched, I could see he was dragging a little boy along with him. He must have been intent because he didn't appear to have noticed me looking at him. I saw him pulling out a chair from underneath a table and then, as he sat down, he lifted the boy onto his knee. Even at some distance, I could tell the boy wasn't happy. Not that I understood why. I just thought he might have wandered away from his mother.

Unable to mind my own business, I wandered over and tried to speak to the man, who looked like he was in his late sixties, and was clearly English. What was he doing with this little boy? The child had just told me that he didn't like the man. Just as I was wondering what I could do to help, I saw a woman running over, saying she was the boy's mum and I could go because everything was all right.

Thank God, he's going to be OK, I thought.

He wasn't.

'Bugger off, you!' she spat out. 'It's not girls he wants.'

I was frightened enough to walk away but, being concerned, I turned around to see what was happening. I still didn't understand, not until I saw him hand the woman some money before he turned the struggling boy over, forcing him face down on his lap.

I'm not going to describe the details of what happened here only to say that it was something so distressing I wanted to scream out loud. Let's just say that after a few minutes the man grunted with pleasure and the little boy, tears running down his face, struggled up on his feet again, spitting out whatever was left in his mouth. That's when I took to my heels and ran back into the bar.

I just about threw myself onto Rob, weeping. I must have stuttered out what I had just seen and heard. He told me there was nothing he could do and that no, the police would not come searching for the man.

'Now I'm going to take you back to the hotel,' he told me firmly. 'You mustn't wander around in the dark, especially in this town.'

I still see that little boy sometimes in my dreams, hear him asking me to help him, and then I hear that mother of his telling him to shut up and do what the nice man wants.

Afterwards, she had shouted at the snivelling child, telling him to shut up and wipe his face.

What happened to him? It is a question that every so often pops up in my mind.

I can only guess.

That's the last memory of my time there.

30

It was Dad who took me to the airport. He had no idea about what happened during my last night and I never told him. He said his farewells to me brusquely after helping me get my luggage checked in. For the first time in my life I was travelling alone. I should have thought that was a bit of an adventure. It might have been if I hadn't been feeling so down. I made every effort to give Dad a cheerful good-bye and thank him for the holiday, but he just nodded his acceptance of these words, pointed out the departure gate and walked away, leaving me to go through security and passport control on my own. I looked back once but he was nowhere to be seen and I was just looking at a wall of Thai faces waving fond farewells to their loved ones. It was not until I was on the plane and fastened my seatbelt that I realised that I had to accept that I no longer had a dad who cared for me. I had got over that once before but getting over it twice when I had held such hopes for the holiday was much worse somehow. I wish I could have ordered some alcohol when the drinks trolley came round, but they knew I was underage so I had to look on as the other travellers poured wine and spirits into their little plastic cups.

I'll have to wait till I'm back in the UK, I told myself.

I had taken my methadone before I left but, unfortunately, it no longer made me feel sleepy and my mind kept replaying the whole holiday as I tried to make sense of my situation. The information that Chelsea had given me about Dad and Dang kept whirling through my head. I now knew that Dad would end up living in Thailand and it was unlikely I would ever be invited out there again for a visit. No wonder he had been generous with money ever since Mum died. It must have been partly so that he could get me out of the way and then later, when he believed he needed me, to help Dang get her UK visa.

I can remember all those lonely days when my younger self came back from school to an empty house where there was no one to welcome her. No comforting smells of home-cooked meals and no hugs as she was asked about her day. How she had to order takeaways because her dad seldom cooked a meal for them and, when he did, it was a ready meal or out of a tin. And how, even if he was in the house, she sat there in silence with no one to talk to. Then there was my breakdown. Even if that boy had not screamed at me, I should think that I might still have collapsed eventually and little wonder if I had. And on that plane journey home I was yet again experiencing the loss of a parent. Only this time I was about to discover that I would not get the help that I had received before.

I wondered if Dad was going to buy a house over there and invest his money in some kind of business. From what I had seen of Dang, I expected that she would try and persuade him to do just that. So, would he sell both of the houses I now knew he owned? If Mum had had a clue that she was going to die young, she would have left me her share of the house, as well as her jewellery. I'm sure she just hadn't thought she was of an age to make a will, but then sudden death is hardly predictable.

Where was I going to live? It was another question churning in my head. I didn't think that Anne would want me to stay with her indefinitely, even though she and Mum had been such good friends. Her two sons currently had to share a bedroom so that I had a room to myself. I had heard the elder one grumbling about it and Anne explaining that they had to be generous because I needed to stay there until my father had returned to the UK and then his brother could have his own room back. But that was before she heard that he had married Dang. She must have been relieved when it appeared that he and I were on good terms again. I'm sure when I went on that holiday, she had her fingers crossed that Dang and I would become so friendly that Dad would bring her to England and we would all live in the house, together.

She was in for quite a shock when she heard about what was really goin on.

The other question that came popping into my head was, why hadn't one of my aunts taken me in after Mum died? Apart from the odd visit to them, they had almost disappeared from my life. *They had their own families who they wanted to spend time with and now that their sister was dead, I was no longer part of their lives*, I thought miserably. With thoughts like these bouncing around in my head, I didn't sleep for most of that flight and, by the time my feet were back on British soil, I felt increasingly down.

Would Anne be waiting for me at the airport? I wondered, hopefully.

No, she wasn't. Dad had clearly forgotten, or perhaps he hadn't bothered, to let her know the time I would be landing. Or maybe he expected me to sort myself out; after all, there were trains and buses. I could have got a taxi as he had put a reasonable amount of money in my bag. I think that must have been one of the last times my younger self was sensible. She decided it would be a lot cheaper if she caught a train and then got a cab for the short journey to Anne's house.

It seemed to take ages to get to Nuneaton and, by the time I arrived and almost crawled into a cab from the station, I was too exhausted to give the driver coherent instructions.

I was slightly worried that Anne might be out, as I had left my keys with her. Luckily, she wasn't. When I arrived, I had to knock on the door. She opened it almost straight away. To me, she didn't seem as warm and friendly as she had always been. No hugs or 'don't you look good?' Instead, she just said, 'Come in, Amy.'

She didn't say anything to me about being worried about me staying with them, but it was easy to pick up the feeling that they certainly didn't want it to go on for much longer. It wasn't only about the space and the boys having to share a room, but also some rumours she heard about from her sons of which I was unaware then. They had said I mixed with bad people; that I went to a house after school where there was a bunch of drinkers and junkies. The woman who lived in the house was middle-aged and known in the town for being an oddball alcoholic. Not only that, her son and his friend, who I had been seen with, were into car theft and drugs.

Looking back now as a mother myself, I suppose it didn't make a case for me being an innocent teenager who needed her help and protection any longer. I suspect she might have searched my room too on hearing these rumours. It was a good thing that I had stopped taking heroin, or I think they would have had me placed in some sort of foster home as fast as they could, but she found a few of my methadone tablets and the prescription. As it was signed by a doctor, I don't think she really knew what the tablets were for, at least not then anyhow, although she did later.

I think now that Anne was hoping that my visit to Thailand might have made a difference to the life I had been living outside both my home and her own. A life that I had kept secret from her. She understood that loneliness can cause someone of my age to mix with the wrong people. On the other hand, since I had been staying with her and had been made to feel such a part of her family, she could ask herself why I had continued behaving that way.

It must have been a couple of days later before Dad contacted Anne to let her know that his house was going up for sale. Yes, he would have to come back in the next couple of months, but only for a short while, to pack it up for good. He gave her a message to give to me: I was to take what I wanted from the house, things like framed photographs, and then I must pack all my own stuff that I had left there before the estate agent arrived to value the place.

I'm sure that's when Anne began to panic. Her eldest son was becoming increasingly vocal about wanting his room back. Not only that, but she also had doubts about me mixing with her boys, especially as she was already thinking I could be a bad influence on them.

The good side of her, the one which was my mother's best friend, wanted me to go back to school and do well, whereas the bad side of me wanted to wreck the house. Thankfully, my good side stopped me from doing that. Besides, there were all the photos of Mum that I wanted to have, though I was much too blind-sided, hurt and confused to think of much else worth having straight away.

Don't be stupid, I told myself, *there are loads of things he won't want. There are all the cassettes with Mum's favourite music you like so much, so take them and the cassette player as well and anything else you fancy.* There was nothing that interesting apart from baking and cooking utensils in the kitchen and they would instantly remind me of Mum so I stopped thinking about it to block out the pain. To be fair to Anne, she let me know that she had told Dad that he would have to wait until the weekend for me to sort everything out.

Somehow I managed to get through school where everyone seemed to think that I had been lucky getting time off to go on holiday. I suppose it must have looked like that on the surface. Then one of the senior girls – Donna – came up and asked me when I would like to meet up at Jacqui's.

'Next week', I told her without saying that I didn't want to give Anne an excuse about staying out yet and I was still too tired from the jet lag anyhow. But it was great seeing some of those friends again.

Once school finished, I took myself off to the clinic to get my new prescription.

The doctor was there when I walked in.

'So how did Thailand go? You're looking healthy,' he told me.

'And how are you getting on with the methadone now? It's been quite a few weeks that you've been taking it.'

I wasn't going to tell him about all the times I had yearned for my old friend or how, especially when I was unhappy, I missed that special buzz that took away the pain. Instead, I simply said, 'I took my tablets each day. They're working all right for me.'

He smiled and gave me another prescription. The one warning he gave me that day was to be careful who I let know about me taking it – 'Some people still see it as a drug.'

'It is, isn't it?'

'Yes, in a way it is, but the idea of having it prescribed is that it will stop you taking the dangerous stuff again. In time, you'll be able to start coming off it.'

After that I went to the chemist and tucked the medication deep in my satchel – I didn't want Anne to see it. She seemed pleasant enough when I got back to the house and remained like that for the rest of the week. Come the weekend, she drove me down to Dad's house so that she could help with my packing.

So, I did as I had planned when I was inside the house but I can't tell you how sad being there was and, as I began to pack up my belongings, I grew very tearful. There was hardly a square inch of that house that did not remind me of Mum and the happy times when she was alive. I put all the cassettes and the cassette player into a box, took down all the photos of Mum from the walls, packed up the last of my clothes that still fitted me, then told Anne I was ready to leave.

'If there's anything you want, better take it now,' I told her. 'Dad's unlikely to keep anything that's here, apart from his clothes, is he?'

'No, I suppose not. He's sending in a cleaner on Monday, that's all I know. There's some good cooking equipment in the kitchen, but hardly any more room in my house for one more thing,' she said sadly.

What I wanted more than anything after that was to meet up with my friends and go to Jacqui's and get completely smashed. Anything was better than sitting in Anne's house acting as though everything was all right, which it wasn't. I needed to have some fun to rid myself of the huge waves of sadness and the immense loss that I felt. Everything that had happened since I returned from Thailand made me picture how my life had been before Mum died; it was the love not only of one parent but of two that I missed so very badly.

It only took me until the Tuesday to arrange to meet up with Donna again and go to Jacqui's. There was always that good old excuse that I was seeing a friend or that I was staying with one so that we could do our homework together that I expected Anne to accept. Only this time there was no 'have a

good time and I'll see you later' type of response, just a quiz-
zical and rather suspicious look. But then I still didn't know
what her sons had told her about the rumours.

31

What made me see Pete again? Didn't I know he was the one who had made me an addict, or was I still refusing to accept that? Looking back, I still remember how unhappy my younger self was. She had believed that her father was taking her on holiday because he still loved her and she had felt so happy at the prospect. She was so glad that he had helped her come off heroin and obtain the methadone and that he hadn't seemed angry with her. When she realised his selfish reason for taking her over to Thailand with him, she was completely shattered.

Even now I still feel a little of the hurt that his actions generated. As my younger self wrote in her diary, 'It's hope that destroys us.' All those dreams of bonding with her father again were snatched from her, shattered into little pieces, the result being she almost completely destroyed her own young life.

It was the loneliness I had felt after Thailand; the realisation that there was no one I could share my feelings with, no one who would understand how I felt, that drew me back to my old ways. The biggest problem was that I could see that my father had done his best to obliterate his memories of my mother. He didn't want me to talk about her either. Not only that, but he clearly had no interest in the daughter they had produced, even though he had once been happy to have me as part of his family. That was then. I knew he no longer wanted any reminder of the past, he was only interested in his future with Dang and there was no place for me.

* * *

When Pete heard I was back, he didn't wait long to turn up at Jacqui's and he certainly used all the charm he could muster that evening on me. He must have known that any feelings I had for him initially were no longer there. As cool and calm as I tried to appear when I was at Jacqui's, beneath all the teenage bravado I attempted to project I was angry with the world. Pete might have been known as the bad boy but that was something I didn't care one iota about. Like him or not, I felt he was someone who understood me. As well as that, he seemed genuinely pleased to see me.

However, I did feel, especially by the way that he reminded me about the time when we had first spoken to each other, that I should not forget how he had lifted my hair out of my face as I vomited. Did he want me back in his life? He looked so relaxed and charming when I laughed a little at that memory.

He chatted away to me, ignoring everyone else and asking me all about Thailand.

'So, Amy, what have you got planned now that you're back?'

'Nothing much,' I answered, 'just catching up with some of my schoolwork.'

A bit later, he invited me out for a meal.

'Do you think you'd like some more Thai food after your holiday? I thought we could go and eat on Friday. You'll be the one who knows their way round the menu this time! Then you have the whole weekend to catch up on your homework.'

It didn't take me more than a few seconds to agree. I did like the restaurant that he and I had been to before and I desperately needed some fun. Besides, what else was I going to do?

'Good! I'll drive you back to Anne's afterwards so that you're not too late getting in. Don't want to annoy her, do you?'

I was pretty sure I already had.

All I told Anne was that a friend was taking me out for a meal. A Thai one, seeing as I'd enjoyed that type of food so much when I'd been there.

'I'll be getting a lift home afterwards,' I told her, not realising this was a mistake. Saying I was out with someone who could drive was telling her that I was going out with someone older than me. Her lips pursed a little when she asked what time I was likely to come back.

'Oh, we'll be going out early, so I'll be back before nine,' I told her quickly, causing her to look a little relieved.

I noticed that she didn't ask me who I was going out with. As I found out later, she already had a suspicion that it was Pete.

* * *

We did have a good time in the restaurant. Pete made sure that whatever he had to say was interesting and he could also make me laugh. Not that I can remember much of the conversation, but I do remember the food: it was good. For once, I was sensible enough only to drink one glass of wine. I knew, as she had asked what time I would be back, it was likely that Anne would be looking out for me when I came in. It was so different from when I had been living in Dad's house. Either he would still have been out with his mates, or already in bed, snoring his head off after having one too many. Whatever it was, it meant that I had no problem sneaking back in late and getting myself into bed. If in the morning he was up as the same time as me, there were seldom any questions asked. He hardly ever asked about my school marks or whether I had homework either. Being at Anne's was not so easy. If I stumbled in smelling of alcohol, she would hardly have been pleased.

Pete acted the perfect gentleman when we walked back to his car. No stopping and trying to attempt a snogging session, thank goodness. Anyhow, I had to look as though all I'd been up to was having an early-evening meal with a friend. Since he met me again at Jacqui's after my holiday, he had acted as though I was just a friend whose company he liked. Silly me, I believed him. He even opened the car door for me before driving me back to Anne's.

That was smart of him, not wanting me to get me into any trouble. I did think for one moment that he was planning to try and get me back and that he believed he could manage this if he went slowly to rebuild my trust, which he managed to do up to a point. We met casually a few times after school, going to the coffee place we had visited before, then I went back to Anne's. A couple of weeks later he told me his parents were away for the weekend. Naturally, he invited me up to his room, but this time it was only to be during the evening.

'We can have a takeaway pizza and listen to music,' he told me. 'Then I'll take you back to Anne's again.'

Again, there was no mention of me staying the night, which would have meant that I would have to think of a really strong excuse to give to Anne.

I said no to changing my methadone for anything stronger after he asked me if it was working well. As the blues played softly in background, I sipped a little wine and tucked into the pizza he had ordered.

Looking back, I can now see the real Pete. Sad it took me too long to recognise it. What I didn't know was that he had studied me enough to know that I was not completely in control of myself. I had told him how I was unable to talk about Mum with Dad, which I found painful, and now at Anne's, I daren't mention the methadone I was taking – I dreaded the thought of her finding out the reason I had been prescribed it. She would then know that I had been taking heroin while under her roof and I could only imagine just how angry that would make her if she learnt what it was for because then she would know I had been addicted. Already she had asked me if I had gone to the doctor to get anything for depression, which is what she might have thought that my script was for.

'Only before I went to Thailand,' had been my answer, which made me wish I could tell her the truth, but I understood that was impossible.

I began to believe that Pete was the only one who would understand what I was feeling. He listened quietly when I told him about the methadone and how I didn't want to go back to heroin. All the while he must have sat there weighing up the chances of getting me, to take it again. Why? Because that would make me dependent on him. He nodded his head, ostensibly agreeing with me and his warm smile made me believe that he was on my side. I didn't have a clue that he was playing along because he wanted to discover exactly what my weaknesses were and knew how to encourage me to tell him more. He made himself out to be a sympathetic listener who wanted to help me get over my problems.

When I said more than once that I wanted to stay on methadone, it told him that I was finding it difficult not to ask him for heroin.

'Good for you, Amy,' was his reply each time and then he frowned a little before saying, 'I understand that you'd like to feel that buzz again, wouldn't you?'

Somehow I stopped myself from saying I would – I so wanted to feel happy again and just one jab could take away all my unhappiness. Instead, I told him as firmly as I could that I wanted to be a normal teenager and not an addict again.

Firm as I thought I was being, Pete wasn't about to give up.

* * *

Not long after that, Dad came back. He more or less ignored me when he came round to Anne's, just handing me an envelope with some money inside.

'Make it last,' he told me.

There would not be much more coming in my direction, I thought. More than likely there would be enough to help me finish my basic education and some sent to Anne but nothing else offered after that. I asked Anne if Dad had said anything to her about helping me once I had finished school or if he still wanted me to go on to further education once I had taken my final exams.

'No, he didn't mention anything like that. He's offered me money for you to stay with me until you finish school, that's all,' she told me flatly.

It didn't take a mind reader to tell me that she was no longer happy with having me in her house. After all, it was supposed to be a temporary situation, not something that could go on indefinitely. I could tell the rest of her family all felt the same way.

It was her husband, Martin, who began asking me questions such as, 'Have you thought of what kind of job you want to do when you leave school?' That was all very well, but I still didn't know then if I was expected to leave school at sixteen or whether Dad was going to help me go on to further education. The trouble was that I hadn't really thought about my future. I might have had dreams of doing something that was quite unlikely, but I had no real plans in my head. And if my mum hadn't died, I'd have been discussing my plans with both of them, which made me feel even worse.

'Wouldn't Dad get me somewhere to live?' I wanted to know.

Then I saw from the way they were looking at each other that this was unlikely.

'You would have to ask him yourself, Amy,' was all they said, which surely meant that they didn't think he had any plans for me.

'Maybe you could train as a hairdresser, seeing you're so good with yours,' Martin suggested with a friendly smile.

'Or you could get a receptionist job at a country hotel, where you could live in,' Anne added.

'Anyhow, have a think about it,' Martin told me quite nicely.

Then I heard Anne say, 'I hope you're working hard at your homework when you and whoever your friend is do some work together.'

From the tone of her voice, I could tell that she didn't believe the excuses I made for not coming straight home from school. As she never asked, I didn't tell her that if I was visiting Jacqui's for the evening and I did my homework there almost as soon as I arrived. Also, if I was out on a Friday night, I caught up with my school work over the weekend.

I don't think either Anne or Martin believed back then that I was doing my best to do everything right. Although I wasn't tempted to take other drugs, I made sure that I only took my methadone. I worked hard at school and every day I was able to hand my homework in, which mostly got me good marks, although my spelling was, and still is, a bit of a problem.

I feel now that as Anne and her husband were adults and

I was still only fourteen, it would have been better if they had sat me down and asked some questions, such as who it was that I did my homework with. I could have told them that it was Donna, a senior girl, who I was able to get help from when I was at Jacqui's. As for Jacqui, she was a middle-aged woman with a young daughter I was really fond of. Was I meeting up with a boyfriend? would have been their first question, I'm sure, and I was surprised they never asked me outright about Pete, given they knew about his reputation. Had Anne asked me about the methadone because she had seen the script, I would have found the courage to tell them why I was taking it. None of that happened, though, and I'm sure they carried on assuming that I must be up to no good.

What adults often don't seem to realise – and I'm speaking from experience here – is that, if they assume the teenager in their care is up to no good, they have an indignant youngster on their hands. One who is likely to make their suspicions come true.

It was Pete who put the most unsuitable ideas in my head, though I must admit I didn't dismiss them altogether, which, let's face it, I should have done. I could get some excitement in my life as well as some money if I joined the gang that he had working with him. A couple in the group were car thieves while the others were the ones who just broke into cars and pinched the stereos or anything else that might have been left there.

'They have insurance,' Pete kept telling me about the car owners. 'They'll get the money to buy new stuff.'

Even now I can't understand why I let myself join that

group. I suppose it was partly because I was depressed and partly because, the way Pete described it to me, it sounded exciting. But I can understand a little why I let him give me heroin again. Which is not to say that I'm not still angry with my younger self for allowing herself to say yes when it was offered. To be fair, I know she was in a dark place then and her energy to fight temptation had been eroded by her feeling unwanted. At the time I didn't stop to think what I needed to do to have a decent future, nor did I realise that I was the one destroying myself.

I was caught in possession of drugs twice but, thanks to my solicitor's convincing plea to the magistrate, I was let off. The third time, I was called up to magistrates' court. Everything changed for me that day, and in a way, I now think it was for the better.

32

Addiction is a poison, or maybe we should call it a virus, because it's not only the user who becomes infected, it's everyone else in their life. It took a long time for my younger self to come to terms with this. Even so, her life remained a struggle and it took several years of summoning up every atom of her guts and determination to walk away from the people who were trying to destroy her. Some of my worst memories are of this time, especially the next part of my life. Let's start with how my family had to step in, but would soon find out that in many ways it was too late.

What was the main reason why I didn't take heed of my solicitor's advice? Had I done so, I might not have ended up in court again. I did try a little, but that was before Pete told me he was short of money and now I would have to pay, one way or another, to get my drugs. I wasn't in any fit state to take a trip to the health clinic and plead for another prescription of methadone. So many times I've wished that I had done just that because it would have made such a difference.

If only I had used some of Dad's money wisely instead of doing what Pete told me to do, maybe my future might have been different.

Instead of doing the sensible thing, I listened to Pete and went back to work with the gang. At least neither Mum's friend Anne nor my Aunt Janet knew I was working with them. I know now that they were horrified when they eventually learnt the truth. When they heard about the court case, they probably thought that I was involved in those petty crimes because I wanted to impress the type of older friends I was mixing with, trying to find the connections I'd sadly lost.

It was Janet, who apart from Dad was my closest relative, who was informed by Jeremy of my arrest and the impending court case, just weeks away. He told her that he was going to try and get me put on probation, which he thought would be a good deal better for me than a custodial sentence. Janet was appalled that her sister's child could be sent to prison but Jeremy did his best to reassure her as he explained his strategy, although he warned that he could not promise the outcome – it was all dependent on the magistrate. Even if he failed, as I had not done anything that serious, I should not receive a sentence longer than a few months. He then asked my aunt if he could state that I would be staying with her until the court case, thereby getting me off the streets and out of any more mischief. Not that he believed I would, I'm sure, but the court had to be completely assured of my wider family's support.

Janet agreed to this and was then saddled with the awkward task of phoning Anne to explain why I would be going to stay with her. She would drive down and collect me the following day. In the meantime, Anne was asked to make sure I didn't go out on my own. The news hardly caused a good atmosphere in the house, although I'm sure Anne and her husband must have been relieved that I would be leaving and no longer their responsibility. You can imagine what they thought about it all. I was convinced they did not want their children mixing with me after they had all their suspicions confirmed. I think they must have sent the boys to stay at a friend's house on my last night there. All I was told was to sort out my packing and not to forget my schoolbooks. It was a good excuse to spend most of my time in my room as the atmosphere was tense.

In a way, I was pleased it was Janet's house that I would be staying at. She was the aunt I had known best, although when Mum was alive. I was very fond of Janet – I had always looked forward to her visits to our house – only this time I dreaded what her reaction would be when we met. I didn't think for one moment that I was going to meet the smiling aunt I had always known, but rather one who was furious at what I had been getting up to.

I felt a little better when she arrived at Anne's home and gave my shoulder a light squeeze. After telling me she had to talk to Anne, she entrusted me with her car keys – 'You can put your luggage in the boot, then just wait for me in the car – I won't be long.'

I'm guessing she had a cup of tea with Anne, said whatever she wanted to say and then heard the worst. What she didn't want to know was that Anne and her husband would never have me back, even if I got off. Not that I knew that then.

33

The following day, Janet's children – my cousins – were at school and then they were spending the evening with friends because my two other aunts had also been summoned to the house. Talk about the going getting tough. The worse line they shot at me, which in one way or another was repeated by each of them in turn, was, 'Thank God your mum isn't here, she would be so ashamed of you.' That was bad enough and really hit home but then came a few more similar ones, which made me cry when I was finally on my own in my room. But when I was with my aunts and those words were slung at me, all I wanted to shout back in my defence was that, if Mum hadn't died and Dad hadn't just abandoned me, then I would never have ended up in this mess. In retrospect, I think they must have been all too aware of this, but their hands were tied in what they could do to help me.

It took a few days for me to tell myself that maybe I could not always use the excuse that my mother dying four years ago had turned me into a thief. 'Thief' being a word that already made me cringe. Janet must have told her sisters about the methadone – Jeremy had no option but to let her know. He had given me a few days' medication, but the rest was handed to my aunt when she visited him before coming to collect me. At least they didn't use the word 'heroin' – they knew, though.

I know now why they were so angry with me: they wanted me to feel ashamed because, if I didn't begin to feel that way and became resentful of the slippery slope that Pete had led me on, they were convinced that there was little chance of me getting my life on a more positive track.

Looking back, I'm sure that their sternness and the difficult questions they threw at me did do me some good. As the days drew closer to the court case, I could only hope that my solicitor would succeed in getting me on probation. The day of the hearing arrived all too quickly. I remember us leaving at the crack of dawn as the car journey was a long one and I sat in the back, sick with nerves. We stopped for breakfast, but I had little appetite and then in, what seemed like no time at all, we had arrived at the court. Now it was time for me to walk to where Jeremy was waiting for me.

My future lay in his hands.

34

That day, as I walked into court for the third time running, I was still hoping that I would be let off. Jeremy was such a good defence solicitor, which made me feel that I might be in luck. A feeling that dissolved the moment my eyes set on the magistrate who was going to deal with my case. While waiting to be taken into the court, I was still pretty certain that I would be leaving by the front door. All I had to do at the end of my short trial would be to swear that I would not break any laws again. That promise would be a sincere one. I had promised everyone, including myself, that I would turn over a new leaf. Then I would be free to go, wouldn't I?

What my younger self hadn't admitted, even then to herself, was that she had become far too confident in committing those little crimes of hers: ones that would make the magistrate lack any sympathy. I listened to all the evidence about me breaking into cars and stealing people's stereos. The last time I had been caught sounded bad, even to me. There were already two stereos in a bag next to my feet when I broke into the gold-coloured Mercedes.

I could picture that evening when the police car pulled up beside the Mercedes. There were hardly any excuses I could use – I could hardly have said what I thought, which was that the owner had to be a rich guy who would hardly miss having to buy a new stereo. At least that's what I had told my conscience, though I'm not sure if I had much of one during those few months. Whatever I stole was handed over to Pete, who occasionally gave me cash, although usually it was the drugs I craved that were slipped into my outstretched palms. The one thing I refused to do was to steal anything personal. If a briefcase or a coat slung over the back seat had been left in a car, I ignored it. This was something I told my solicitor and something he checked up on: 'You told me the truth, Amy. All the complaints about the stereos being stolen did not include anything else.'

At first, I wasn't that short of cash – Dad had left me some after he sold both his houses and returned to Thailand. I don't know what he said to Anne apart from goodbye. She did tell me that he had arranged to send her some money each month in return for my keep but that was about all she said. I suppose he must have offered a reasonable amount. Still, I was upset that the woman who had been so kind to me then was no longer happy having me in her home, even if I understood why.

So, what excuse can I give for breaking the law? I guess I did it to fit in with the other thieves who worked around Pete and also to feed my habit. Not that those were good excuses, were they? But they were the only ones I had.

The one thing I finally learnt while I was in prison was that drugs might take away sad memories, but they also quietly remove most of our common sense. In my case, let's face it, there was hardly a scrap of it left in my head. Previously when I had been in court, the magistrate appeared to feel sorry for me. He gave me a bit of a ticking-off, followed by some advice not to get into trouble again and then I was set free.

Even my solicitor was surprised at that. I could tell by the expression on his face as we left the court that he had not agreed with how the magistrate had spoken to me at the end. A good warning, telling me firmly that this would be the last time I would leave by the front door, might have been more appropriate.

Jeremy took me to a coffee shop after my case wrapped; he clearly wanted to talk to me. He told me that I had been extremely lucky, 'So please, Amy, don't get yourself back in the magistrates' court again. You'll not get off for a third time. It will be prison for you and you won't like it. And think a little about your relatives and Anne too – they would be shocked if they knew all about this. I should have informed them and, if you get into trouble again, I will, especially if you're charged again. Because if you are, it will not end well.'

I should have listened to him then and turned over a new leaf straight away, shouldn't I? But no, of course, I didn't. Which is why I was finally looking at a stern-faced magistrate whose eyes bore into mine with such distaste.

* * *

I had made myself look as neat and tidy as I could for my third appearance in court. My aunts had instructed me to wash my face clean of make-up, not to wear nail varnish and to scrape my hair back into a neat ponytail. No jeans, they stressed, so taking their advice, I wore my school uniform. When I looked in the mirror, I saw a typical schoolgirl. Jeremy must have been of the same mind as my relatives. On seeing me, he looked surprised. His eyebrows shot up and he said, 'Well done, Amy – you look nice and smart and very appropriate.' Even though he had already warned me that he did not believe I would get off so easily this time, I knew that he hoped that I would be put on probation instead of being sentenced to prison.

I can remember my younger self thinking, *if I look good and innocent then I just might get off.*

She got that wrong.

That day, the magistrate only asked me a couple of questions. I replied as politely as I could not that my answers seemed to sway him in any way at all. From the expression on his face when my solicitor spoke in my defence, no reaction was evident. That was when my heart sank: somehow, I knew my luck had finally run out. I was right, it had.

The magistrate looked at me coldly and called me a habitual thief. I needed to understand how serious my crimes were, he said. He then sentenced me to two years at a young offenders' section of a women's prison. I was sure I heard my solicitor gasp at the severity of the sentence. In his defence speech, he had brought up the fact that I had never stolen anything personal from the cars, which he claimed showed I did have some principles. None of these facts made any impression, it seemed. I guess the magistrate's mind was made up as soon as he knew my past record as well as my present crimes. He went on to say that the institution where he was sending me had strict wardens but very good teachers. That meant I would not miss out on schooling, which might just improve my education and give me an opportunity for a future after prison.

I could hardly bring myself to look over to where Anne and Janet were sitting. They and my other two aunts might have tried to support me during the time between being arrested and going to court, but still I knew underneath that they must be disappointed and angry. Anne certainly had every reason to feel I had been deceitful and dishonest.

It was Janet who came down to my cell to wish me luck in the prison and to say that at least I would get some good schooling while I was there. As I could wear my own clothes, she would make sure that some suitable ones were delivered, plus a few essentials I would need. I was still in shock so I'm surprised I can remember what she told me. Anne then came to say goodbye and I could tell by the tone of her voice that this goodbye was final and I would not be going back to her home when I was released. She was only there for a couple of minutes and, when she left, all I could do was sit and wait for the warden to come and take me to the prison.

It seemed a long time before I was escorted into what looked like a large van. The warden snapped the handcuffs on me as I walked out of the magistrates' courts. This time, as Jeremy had predicted, it was the back door I was walking out of. I noticed the windows were blacked out, presumably to stop people looking in. Within minutes I was being driven through the town. Going through it like that made me think how I had been free to walk the streets for years. It would be a long time before I would have that freedom again; tears were beginning to prickle. *Don't let them*, I told myself firmly and so I did my best to swallow them down. It was my fault that I was where I was now and, in a way, that made it even harder.

The drive from the court to the prison was not long. As we drew closer, I could see that all around the prison were farms and fields, which looked beautiful to me. It was when the van drove through the huge green metal gates and I heard them slamming shut that I felt terrified – it was as if I had entered another world from which there was no escape.

Don't show any weakness if you don't want to be bullied, my inner voice snapped at me. That made me sit up as straight as I could. I was seated with other new arrivals all around the same age as me while the wardens sorted out our registration. A couple of them were laughing and joking as though they were happy to be there – it seemed this was not the first time they had been sent to prison. The others looked as miserable as I felt and, though I was curious about my fellow inmates, I couldn't bring myself to say a word.

The next stage was having our mugshots taken and filling in forms about our medical histories, which was not too bad. But the last one was. Although we were allowed to wear our own clothes and not uniforms, that did not stop the wardens from searching our clothes and, even worse, our bodies. They were looking for drugs, phones and weapons, such as knives or razor blades. Afterwards we would be permitted to have a shower. That final strip search was thoroughly degrading. I was told to remove every item of clothing and then to go behind one of the screens that had been put up, where a warden would check me. I had to keep turning different parts of my naked body until I was told to squat down so my intimate parts could also be checked.

It must have been about three hours before every procedure in those rooms had been carried out. After the shower when I was handed back my clothes, the warden said she could see I had a drugs problem. I looked at her, wondering why she had said that. Seeing the look on my face, she simply said, 'I've seen those marks on your body. That tells me.'

'I've been taking methadone for a while,' I told her.

'Then you will have to see the doctor here,' she said.

I was beginning to feel shaky so this came as something of a relief.

At least that was until I heard her final words: 'Oh, sorry, just seen the time. Doctor's gone home now, you'll have to wait till morning.'

What she meant was that I would have to suffer withdrawal symptoms all night.

And so I did.

35

What was my life like in prison? To tell the truth, the young offenders› section was nothing like as bad as I thought it would be. My cell was better than the one I had spent a couple of nights in when I was dragged into the police station. The bed was small, but then so am I. There were even shelves where I could put my books and a small table that I could work on; the food wasn't that bad, either.

But, as you might expect, my first night was miserable. By the time I joined the other girls in the canteen for dinner, my whole body was shaking as I was craving my methadone and I knew that I was going to have a bad night ahead. One of the girls said, 'I can see you need your meds. Doctor will be here in the morning, she'll get you sorted out.'

'What's she like?'

'She's OK, quite nice actually.'

Another one chipped in then, saying she, too, had a bad first night when she came in and, like me, had to wait until morning to get meds. It seems like the wardens made sure that, by keeping new inmates in the shower rooms, it was common for the doctor to have left for the day by the time they were ready to see them.

Phew, I thought, *I'm not the only one here who has a habit*. In fact, it turned out that quite a few of the girls had. It didn't take me long to get to know the different ways they had got the money to feed their habit, which led to their incarceration. These crimes were the reason that so many of them were in there.

That evening, I was too strung out to take in much more of the conversation. It was even difficult to swallow the food I had in front of me. As soon as I could, I left the other girls, who were chattering away, and went back to my cell. Sometime later, I heard the cell doors being locked and then the lights went out. It was a sharp shock that made me acknowledge that, even if we could wear our own clothes and have school classes, we were all, nevertheless, prisoners. I lay there in the dark with my body shaking and it felt as though a thousand spiders were crawling over me. That first night I didn't get an inch of sleep.

By the time daylight came and the cell lights went on, I was feeling more than wobbly. For once, I was pleased to see the face of authority with the arrival of the warden. After unlocking my door, she came in: 'The doctor's arrived. I'm going to take you straight to her.' She wrapped my dressing gown around my heaving shoulders, saying I could get dressed after my meds were sorted out.

The blonde-haired doctor I met just a few minutes later was young and friendly, which was a relief, as I had been expecting someone stern and critical of my drug habit but she was just about the opposite. She smiled at me and told me to sit down, then there were questions about how long I had been taking heroin without sounding in the least bit disapproving. Her only objection was the harm it did to young bodies and the long-term damage it could do.

I told her I had been on methadone for some time and should have stayed on it, but was then tempted to go back onto hard drugs and got caught stealing. All she said was, 'I'll put you on to methadone now. Won't be long for you to feel better.'

She was right – it only took a few days for me to feel a lot calmer. I did sleep a lot, but I still managed to go to classes. I noticed that quite a few girls were not interested, but I was determined to catch up on my education.

When my drowsiness stopped, I got to know quite a few of the girls there. Some were in for what I saw as unpleasant crimes, such as using some kind of weapon to get people to hand over their money. Standing near a cash machine and waiting for a person to draw out money before coming up behind them and demanding the cash as they brandished a knife. These girls were caught acting suspiciously on CCTV; their crime was recorded and replayed in court.

Then there were others whose drug habits made them shoplift. And others so desperate that they sold their underage bodies for a few pounds to men in cars who knew the place where the younger girls were to be found.

At least, I thought gratefully, I had never been so desperate to do that.

One of them had become pregnant after one such encounter, when she had barely turned fourteen. It was her boyfriend who pushed her out onto the streets and he who made her steal as well to support both of their addictions. And even at eight months pregnant, the men still wanted to pay her for sex. Her boyfriend had dumped her at the entrance to the hospital and disappeared. The baby was taken from her and put into care almost as soon as it was born.

There were many more sad stories I heard while I was there. Girls whose childhoods had been so terrible that they ran away from their family homes for their own safety. They ended up living in squats with people who had no interest in being law-abiding. I suppose they must have been controlled by people much worse than Pete.

There were a couple of very muscular, tough-looking girls that I was advised to keep away from. They had been violent outside and, now inside, they could really cause damage to the other inmates. These two girls wouldn't have hesitated to use weapons had their victims resisted. The moment I saw them, I instinctively knew they were trouble and took an immediate dislike to them. They were the kind who walk around with clenched fists and only smile if they manage to harm someone else.

The girl in the next cell to me, Sue, was the one I became friendly with during the time we were both there. Almost as soon as I walked onto the wing, I met her. It took a couple of days before we really got to talk – I think she must have waited until the methadone had done its job. She made some flirtatious comments that made me laugh and reply, 'I'm straight,' to which she responded, 'Yeah, that's what they all say.' She laughed along with me before introducing herself. From then on, we spent a lot of time together. Like me, she was keen to get educated and she also wanted to get into rehab. What was she in for? I was never sure. I knew her sentence had been longer than mine, that's all, but I never asked. If people didn't offer it, you just didn't. From the first day we talked, we did just about everything together and it was being with her so much of the time that stopped those bullies coming near me.

* * *

Quite a few of the inmates were wary of Sue. I heard them muttering behind her back that she was a loudmouth who never seemed scared of anything.

'That's bullshit,' I said angrily, 'she's really kind-hearted. And I should know.'

OK, so Sue didn't take any shit. She believed that we all had to stand up for ourselves – a lesson she gave me more than once. 'Those two over there are a real menace,' she told me one day, pointing to the two women I already disliked. 'You be careful, Amy. They steal your things and, if you complain, they beat you up. Just ignore them when you walk past them. Shoulders back and chin up. Got it?'

I got it! I might have been over six inches shorter than them, but I knew how to move fast and, after all I'd been through, it took a lot for girls like that to frighten me. I sensed they were aware of it and left me alone.

It must have been a couple of weeks after I arrived that one of youngest inmates, who was only thirteen, got beaten up badly. Not only was she black and blue, but her card – the one she could make phone calls with – was stolen. We all knew who did it, but she was too frightened to tell. I was shocked, but then I hadn't been there long enough to know that things like that can happen inside.

That night, after it had happened, we were talking through our doors when the alarm went off, which made us all nervous. We could hear the sound of the wardens' boots pounding up the corridors, but no one knew what had happened. The next morning, we learned that the wardens had saved that thirteen-year-old girl's life. Unable to bear the treatment those two heavyweight girls were giving her, she had tried to kill herself. She had pulled the sheet from her bed, tied it to one of the bars of her window and then tied the other part of the sheet around her neck before climbing up onto a chair and jumping off.

I came out of my cell that day as soon as the doors were un-locked and asked Sue if she'd heard what happened. She told me about the girl and it was the look she gave me that said she was going to sort out those bullies. She got into the older one's cell and, before I could stop her, she had kicked her nearly unconscious. She hated bullying, she told me. I thought she would get into trouble, but she didn't. Instead, the two who had beaten up the girl disappeared from our lives within days – I think they must have been transferred to a much-stricter young offenders' institution.

Everyone there must have been relieved to see the back of them.

I knew from the moment Sue and I became friends that, as she had been in there for some time, she would be leaving before me. Six months later, she was released. As we said our goodbyes, we promised to keep in touch and I did my best to cover up how bleak I felt. Don't get me wrong, I was happy for her that she was getting out and going straight to rehab. It meant, as she had always told me, that she was determined to start her life over again. We did stay in touch for quite a long time. I missed her a lot, but I didn't let that stop me from studying as hard as I could. That's how I spent the next few months waiting for my release – working hard and staying out of trouble.

It was something that happened some time after I was released that made me lose touch with Sue. But years later, I found her on Facebook and we were able to tell each other about our journeys to turn our lives around.

A journey that was far from easy for me after I was released.

Although I had been sentenced for two years, I was released a few months earlier for good behaviour. As I was underage, still not yet sixteen years old, I had to move in with a family. The day before I was due to be released, the prison social worker took me to her office so that she could explain a few things about where I would live when I left. I had been hoping that it would be my own family I would go to, but I was not that surprised when I was told that was not going to happen.

It wasn't so much the conviction for theft that had stopped my family from taking me in, it was the drugs. None of my aunts wanted their children to know where I had been or why and these were just some of the reasons the social worker explained to me. She did her best to be as tactful as possible, I give her that, but being told that no one in your family wants anything to do with you hurts, it really does.

I could just imagine them all sitting together, speculating about what sort of people I had been mixing with in prison. Lots of junkies, no doubt. I could hear them in my head saying, 'I expect she made friends with the worst sort. I mean, she didn't have any decent ones outside of prison, did she?' That much was true, I hadn't, as I was about to discover after I was free. Yes, there were quite a few girls who had been on drugs inside, but the aim in there was to make us want to be clean. Not only because once we were inside we had no choice, but also to encourage us to turn our backs on drugs when we left to live in the real world again.

To my family, I guess methadone was a drug – one I would be taking for a long time – and there was every risk I would get back on to the illegal ones too. Yes, I felt like crying when I listened to the social worker. I hadn't had a visitor for several months, although my aunts had occasionally visited me during my first year there. Anne never came once. Janet was the one who brought in certain things that I needed, such as some new underwear and toiletries. But I could tell that she, like her sisters, hated being there. After these visits I used to imagine them rushing home to have a bath after throwing their cloths straight into the washing machine.

I had written to each of them to tell them that I was sorry, because I really was. Prison had taught me a lot, though once I was out, I could truly say that I hadn't been taught enough. My father, who was still living in Thailand and hadn't made a trip over in the time I was put away, had agreed that once I was released I could live with a foster family and; he also asked my social worker to arrange for me to go to a school near my foster family. From what I was told, he had left everything for the social workers to organise as it seemed he had no intention of travelling back to the UK. He had agreed to send me pocket money so that I could buy necessities, I was told.

I almost felt excited at the thought of going shopping again and maybe even treating myself to a coffee and a cake. That idea was quickly removed from my head. I could hardly believe it when the social worker explained that none of the cash would be given directly to me: 'Your dad has insisted on that. Carol, the woman you will be staying with, will be in charge of it. If you need anything, you will have to ask her to get it for you.'

I could feel my eyes smarting with tears of humiliation. How could Dad not even let me have some pocket money? Determined not to show how upset I was, I fought to choke back those tears.

'Now, a little bit of good news, Amy,' the social worker continued. 'Your Aunt Janet has given me a parcel with some new underwear and a few other things for you to have when you leave here.'

The only thing wrong with having a couple of large carrier bags with some new clothing inside was that they had been handed to the social worker and not me. Still, I had to feel a little pleased that, after being in the prison for well over a year, I would have some decent-looking clothes to wear once I was out.

'As you have done well at school in here,' the social worker went on, 'your father has also stated that, should you want to take some courses when you finish school, he will support you. The teachers here have written a letter saying you worked hard and that they wish you well when you leave.'

That touched me. Their belief in me made me tell myself that, if I did well at the outside school and ended up in a good job, I should be able to become friendly with my family again. There were times over the months and years of my struggles that I had tried so hard to live a normal life yet still my inner voice piped up, *Why do you want to?*

I understood from the one letter Dad had sent me while I was in prison that he would give me help until I turned eighteen. After that I would have to be in control of my own life. Passing my GCEs now became a focal part of my ambitions for my future.

If only I could have seen what lay ahead, I would have committed some stupid crime before my release. Nothing too serious, but enough to alter the plans for my release. Had I remained at the young offenders' institution longer, it would have been a much safer place than the one I was going to.

36

I don't know how many interviews the social workers had with the foster parents that I met the day I left prison. From my point of view, I would say it must have been just one interview and probably one that took as little time as possible. I met other teenagers in prison who had lived in foster parents' homes and, between us, we concluded that not all of them loved children – they just liked the money they were paid for having us. It was those conversations that made me expect that I would be living with a strict couple who would show little warmth or interest in me. But to my relief, that was not the way I saw my foster parents when I first arrived there to stay.

Carol was the one I met straight away. With her short, curly red hair, jeans and baggy shirt, she was a little different from the person I had expected I was going to be living with. The social worker hardly stayed more than a couple of minutes. After telling me to do well, she said her goodbyes and then it was just Carol and me, standing in the large, cosy-looking living room.

'Call me Carol, Amy,' she said with a quick smile. 'I think that will be easier for you.' She went on to tell me that she had put a table in my room so that I could do my homework there – 'We do have a lot of visitors here, so you can escape upstairs whenever you need to, though you are welcome to be with us when your homework is finished.'

Yes, I thought, *I like her*, as I did her husband Martin when I met him later. He was from Jamaica and he told me that his parents had come to England and settled when he was just a baby. Both of them certainly liked playing that country's music, which had a great beat to it. I could hear them laughing as they kept mentioning the words 'pot', 'weed' and 'spliffs' each time Bob Marley's reggae music came on. That was someone I hadn't even heard of before, let alone some of the other artists like the Wailers, Peter Tosh and Marcia Griffiths, but when I listened to their music, I could hardly stay still, which seemed to both amuse and please Martin.

Carol hardly ever tried to act like a strict foster parent. Most of the time I felt she was barely aware that I was there. She knew I was on methadone, mentioned the local chemist where I could take my script (prescription) and gave me the directions so I could find it. I was surprised that neither of them asked any questions about how long I had been on it and they never asked questions about what drugs I had been taking before I was prescribed methadone. I suppose as the doctor at the young offenders' prison had prescribed it, they would know I had been on hard drugs before I went there. Maybe the social worker had already told them all they needed to know. Nor were there any warnings from them to say just how bad it would be for me if I went back on to those illegal drugs. Neither did they ask me anything about my time in prison or why I was not with my father or my aunts. That made me curious, for they were hardly acting like guardians at all.

When I had been there for just over a week, Carol and Martin told me they had a large group of friends coming over on the Saturday.

'Do you mind giving me a hand in the kitchen?' Carol asked me. 'Then you can join us.'

'Of course not,' I said, feeling quite pleased to be included.

The guests who turned up were all men. Nice and friendly enough, but still I wondered why their wives or girlfriends were not with them. I passed around food and chatted to some of them for a while before going up to my room.

I had thought this would be a one-off type of evening, but it turned out that groups of Carol and Martin's friends arrived most evenings. I would be in my bedroom doing my homework when I would hear the doorbell ringing and male voices in the hall, which told me there were people arriving. About an hour later, Carol would call me to say supper was ready and, when I went down, I would meet the friends who were there. Most of them were the men I had met before. They were all welcoming and yet they did not ask me any questions about why I was there. During those weekday visits, I would first eat in the kitchen and then help Carol pass food around to their friends.

Did I enjoy those evenings? Yes, up to a point I did. But after a few times of being with those visitors, I began to feel there was something odd happening. It was the guests that made me feel that way; I couldn't put my finger on it straight away, but I sensed it and this caused questions to start to spin around in my head. There was something about all of them that told me that these were not normal hardworking men, calling in after a full day's work. What did they do to earn a living and why were there no wives or girlfriends with them? I didn't think for one moment that any of them were in highly paid jobs. There was something about them which told me they did not earn their money through working in offices, factories or shops. Nor, from remarks about their cars, did I believe that they were lorry or taxi drivers. So, what did they do? Not that I ever asked, instead, I listened carefully as I tucked away scraps of information in my mind.

My instincts turned out to be correct. It was when I went to one of their parties that I discovered that one of the men, a huge guy called Andy, was a drugs dealer. Or rather, as far as I understand, he was the boss of the group.

I'm convinced that Carol and her husband were aware of where that friend of theirs got his money from. His flashy car stated that he was well off, as did his clothes and those sharp snakeskin shoes of his, and then there were the heavy gold chains round his neck, a huge gold watch on his wrist and a selection of gold rings on his fingers. Surely no one would have thought he had an ordinary job, would they?

Looking back, I soon worked out the reason why Carol and Martin had agreed to have me in the house. They knew all about my past, which told them that I would hardly be shocked if I found out that I was in a world of characters who were actively dealing and run screaming to my social worker.

Plus, I produced a nice little income for them, which went straight into Carol's pocket. I can't say she wasn't generous, though. If I needed anything, she gave me some money and let me do my own shopping, as well as treating myself to that coffee and cake when I was out.

I had told her that I had dreamt of that when I was still inside, which made her laugh.

'You go for it, Amy,' she told me.

During the four months I lived with them, their house was nearly always full of 'friends' and even more seemed to turn up over the weekends. One did tell me that he worked on the door of a nightclub, which I knew was a polite way of saying that he was a bouncer. Another mentioned something about his business without describing what it was.

Now I'm fairly certain that a bouncer can sell a lot of drugs to the youngsters coming into the clubs and the way they interacted with each other told me that all these men were part of the 'business'.

Andy had a certain charm – crooks, I have learnt, often do. He was friendly and chatted to me quite often, telling me about his wife and his two children. He was the only one I ever asked why his wife wasn't ever with him.

'Because we can't leave the kids alone, now can we?' he said firmly, giving me a look that stopped me saying something like, 'Haven't you heard of babysitters?' If he wanted to use his children as an excuse for going solo, then I knew it would be best to mind my own business.

I was surprised when, on the last Saturday I stayed with them, Carol and Martin told me that I was invited to go to a

BBQ with them. Grateful for anything to relieve the boredom of spending the day on my own, I agreed to go. A warm day for once, I had a good reason to wear some of my clothes that looked more like summer holiday ones. On went a pair of leggings and a baggy, shocking pink T-Shirt. My hair, which was now halfway down my back, was tied back in a neat ponytail and I applied a small amount of make-up.

I was hoping that I would meet some other teenagers there and have some fun. On arrival, I could see the garden was packed with lots of people who, like Martin, were mainly West Indian. Music was playing through large speakers and, as I walked up to them, I could see a trestle table laden with lots of drink. For the first couple of hours, I was enjoying myself – I drank some of the rum and sampled some delicious spicy food, many dishes totally new to me. The music made my body move and I loved the reggae sounds.

All around me were men who were going back and forth to help themselves to drinks. As they gathered around the table, I felt their eyes on me. It was then I began to feel uncomfortable – I didn't know everyone and there was hardly any one of my age group there.

It was Andy who came over to me. 'You're looking a little wasted, Amy,' he told me and offered to drive me home if Martin and Carol didn't want to leave yet. He walked over to them with me and, when I told them I was feeling tired and he would give me a lift, Carol just fumbled in her handbag and passed a key to me. Clutching the spare house key, I got into his car.

I know now that this should never have happened. Foster

parents should never let a slightly inebriated fifteen-year-old girl get into a car with a man whose reputation was hardly a good one. What I concluded was that they never wanted to argue with him, although they could have said that they were just about to leave as well and prevented the whole thing.

The drive should have been a short one and for a while I thought that Andy must know a different route until he slowed down as we came to a wooded area. It was when he pulled over in a quiet and secluded spot and I saw the lecherous expression on his face as he looked over at me that I felt frightened.

'Why are we stopping?'

'Think you know why,' he told me.

Then, when I tried to open the car door and found it was locked, I was even more scared. I heard him snigger at that. He leant towards me and the next thing was me feeling the seat being pushed back flat – I think I was just about terrified by then. He was such a big man and I knew I couldn't fight him off.

He began stroking my face and I yelled at him to stop. 'Shush now, Amy,' he said as his face came over mine, causing me to take in his foul breath. His fat fingers held my neck, which forced me to keep still.

'You open your legs for me and I'll give you the drugs you like so much,' he told me. 'I've plenty in my house.'

I tried to shake my head until I felt those fingers of his tighten.

'I know you're a little junkie,' he whispered in my ear, which made me cringe. 'Heard you sold that puny body of yours for drugs.'

I just about managed to spluttered out an indignant denial.

He shook me by my neck then. 'Dirty little junkies always lie,' he hissed. 'So don't try and tell me you've not screwed around and now you're going to do it again.'

'Please,' I kept saying, 'please don't.'

'I have a little game we can play. I'm going to try and get inside you, but I won't hit you if you try and push me off. So, let's see how this game works, shall we?'

I heard the zip of his trousers coming down, saw one hand reach down to his pocket and take out a condom, which he waved triumphantly in my face.

'Don't want to catch anything from a whore junkie,' he told me.

'No, please don't do this,' I spluttered again, choked with tears and fear.

He was nearly on top of me and, pinned as I was, I could hardly move. I felt his hands pull down my leggings as he rose up a little and then a searing pain as he shoved himself into me with immense force. Huge hands grabbed my breasts and he squeezed them so hard that I screamed with pain. I could hear his breathing getting faster as he pushed and pushed and then, with a load groan, his huge body convulsed and it was over.

That pain was worse than what I felt a few years later when I gave birth to my daughter.

'I'll tell,' I warned breathlessly.

'What, Carol and Martin? They wouldn't dare make me angry. If I want you when I come to their house, they won't stop me doing what I like with you.'

With hindsight, I doubt whether what he told me that day was the truth, but back then my younger self believed him.

'I'll take you back now, you little white junkie whore,' he said as I pulled my leggings back on, anxious to cover up.

One thing I noticed as I bent down to pull them up was a bulging wallet. It must have fallen out of his trouser pocket and I was determined to get hold of it. I used my toes to draw it nearer to my bag that was on the floor at my feet.

How I managed to get hold of it when he was reversing the car, goodness knows, but I did. I pretended I wanted to make myself look tidy as I brought up my bag and took out a comb. At the same time, I slipped the wallet inside.

That was the day I became homeless.

* * *

After he had pulled up at the house to drop me off, I flew inside. Fortunately, Carol and Martin were not home yet. As I stood under the hot shower, I thanked God that at least he had used a condom. Even so, I was falling apart.

You've got to get out of here, my inner voice told me.

I packed as many of my things as I could into my duffle bag, threw the keys through the letter box as I left and then ran as fast as I could.

As I neared the station, I checked the wallet: it was stuffed with large bank notes.

Get on a train and get away from this town, my common sense told me.

Which is exactly what I did.

37

I decided that I needed to phone Carol once I got to the town that I was planning to go to next; somewhere I had never been to before. After all, she had been kind to me and I didn't want to get her in trouble with the social services. No doubt she would have to explain that I had run away while she and Martin were at a party.

Go and find a café and get yourself something to eat, my inner voice told me. *You don't want to be ringing her too soon or she might just check on the train departures.*

It was already growing dark when I found a fast food place and ordered a burger and chips and a chocolate shake. I had enough money to stay there for a while, thanks to the money in Andy's wallet, which I went through carefully while I was sat there. There were other things in it, including a collection of bank and credit cards that made the hairs on my neck prickle. Not only were they from different banks, but they were all in different names. That got my curiosity and made me ferret a bit more. I found a slip of paper which told me about money he had placed in each bank over the last few months. Underneath were a number of ATM slips giving the dates and the amounts he had deposited. He seemed to pay around £2,000 into each of these accounts every week.

Having that information to hand could potentially be dangerous as he would want to find me. Not because of the cash in his wallet, but who I might give that information to. After I had pondered the risks, I decided to ring Carol in the morning instead. I needed to make her think that I had travelled a much further distance than I had. Even if I sent the cards and the slip of paper back, that wouldn't keep me out of danger. I might have wanted revenge for Andy raping me and he knew I had it in my hands. What was to stop me making a list of these things, one that would get the police hammering on his door? No doubt that would wreck the business he was running.

For a few seconds I even considered going to the police. *Don't be stupid*, I told myself. That would tell him which town I was in and give him every reason to seek revenge. He had enough people around him to make sure he would get it too. At that point I began to feel really frightened.

As I sat there wondering what I could do next, I realised it was dark outside. Where was I going to stay? I had planned to book somewhere for a night, a plan that I decided would not work now that I had this evidence of Andy's shady dealings in my hands. As I was young, a cheque book or credit card would raise questions; all his cards said 'Mr' so that wasn't an option. Anyhow, I wasn't foolish enough to use them.

What would happen if Carol had already informed social

services that I had gone missing, as she was obliged to do by law? Maybe they would have already informed the police to tell them that I was a missing child. Which meant that, if a hotel contacted the police, I would be immediately traceable. Those were only some of the fears racing through my mind.

The only thing I could do was wander around and find somewhere to sleep. The wallet was best kept well out of sight, so I went to the loo and slid it into my knickers. I hated the thought of anything of Andy's being near the still-sore and tender place between my legs, so I put the wallet in the back of my knickers near my bottom – I didn't want some other homeless person running their hands through my pockets.

Walk out of the city centre – there are too many clubs where lots of people will be milling around on a weekend night. Find a park, stay in the dark, my inner voice urged. I must have walked around until the town appeared lifeless and then tried to get some sleep on a park bench. It goes without saying that I didn't have a good night – park benches are not the best way to get your beauty sleep!

I phoned Carol in the morning. As she heard my voice, she was just about at screaming point. Yes, she was going to inform social services – she had to. But the most worrying thing was that Andy had been round looking for me: he wanted that wallet back.

Now I'm not a good liar, but that morning I did my best when it came to mixing truth with untruth. The truth was that he had raped me, which was why I had run away. I never wanted to set eyes on him again.

'He didn't!' Carol said feebly, but I knew from her lack of protest that she believed me.

'He did, he really hurt me,' I told her and, as soon as the words were out of my mouth, I could hear Carol's voice choking up with tears.

'He just about pushed me out of the car when we got to your house so how could I have his wallet?'

'Because he never got out of the car, Amy, did he?' she said. 'That's what he told me and you've almost confirmed that. He knew it was in his pocket when he got in the car with you.'

'Well, maybe it fell out of the car when he pushed me out and someone else found it,' I said, hoping she might believe me.

And it seemed she didn't, for her next question was how did I have enough money to travel by train?

'I had a bit saved up,' I said defiantly before kicking myself for not denying that I had caught a train.

She then asked me where I was. I was immediately suspicious. Would she have told him? I don't think so, but I believed that he had power over everyone in their group.

'Best if I don't tell you, isn't it?' I said, while she still tried to persuade me to come back.

According to her, there were many reasons for me to return, such as my schooling, and what about all the things that I had left behind? 'We'll look after you, Amy,' she kept saying, but I was far too scared to agree to go back.

At that point I ended the conversation by hanging up. She might have had some valid arguments but none of them got through to me. It was too dangerous for me to go back. Besides, would social services believe me, a child who had just left prison and who had been addicted to heroin? Most probably not, I thought.

*   *   *

I went shopping that day. The next foolish thing that I did was to buy a new SIM card. I put some of the phone numbers on it. What I didn't think then was that, in chucking my old one away, it meant there was no one who could get in touch with me, unless I phoned them. That included everyone in my family, though I still don't know if they ever tried. I also forgot to place Sue's number on it. Although I knew she was in rehab by then, I could have asked her for help later on.

That day I also bought a blanket and a few other essentials before I went to a charity shop and found just what I needed: a tatty-looking large rucksack, which I could put everything into. *That will do*, I decided, as I walked into a world of loneliness. I just wished I was back in prison. There was no one I could contact who would help me, not now I had been inside. Pete certainly wouldn't want me around – most probably he blamed me for going to court. As for my aunts, I didn't think they ever wanted to hear from me again.

And my father? No chance there.

As my options died, each one rejected by me, my cheeks became wet with tears of defeat and desperation.

I'm not going to describe my life on the streets too much – I expect most people have seen enough rough sleepers in doorways to know what it might be like. I was on those streets for quite a few months. In that time, I was soaked by rain and, one night, I witnessed a drunk vomiting all over a homeless boy. I was also offered money for sex, which I thought was an insult. As my funds diminished, I ransacked food from bins near takeaway places to survive.

It was waking up on Christmas morning that almost broke me. I had found a greenhouse on an allotment to sleep in and, when the early hours came, I could see lights being turned on in the houses opposite. Christmas tree lights twinkled in windows and I could imagine how full of life those homes with children would be. I pictured happy little children having an exciting morning opening presents before the family gathered for a big lunch. Once, I had all that as well. Memories of my childhood when I woke to find a stocking at the bottom of my bed full of presents were a kick in the throat. Honestly, I wouldn't have minded if I had closed my eyes and never woken up again.

Missing family life turned out to be the least of my problems while living on the streets. At night, those who had woken at daylight and tried to sleep straight after nightfall were often attacked by groups of drunks. Thankfully, that never happened to me. Feeling I had no choice, I made myself walk the streets until the early hours before finding a place I felt safe in. There was one spot behind a swimming baths with a heater blowing out warm air, which made the cold nights slightly more bearable.

Over those months, cautious as I was about spending the money from the wallet, it had begun to disappear. No longer able to get methadone, I had found a dealer – another homeless person (they're never that hard to find on the streets)

– who was able to get me my old friend. Once again, I was injecting myself. It was the only way I could cope with the world that I now found myself in. I would rather live in a drug-addled haze than face the reality of my life at that time.

I dread to think how I might have ended up if I hadn't met people from the charities that at night brought us hot drinks and food. It was a lovely couple who saved my life: they saw I was cold and took me to their charity's storeroom, where they found me warmer clothes and a snug pair of boots. They also paid for me to stay in a hostel for a couple of weeks.

'Our daughter was an addict,' the woman told me. 'She's no longer with us. It was heroin that killed her.' They asked me my age and I added on a year – I didn't want the authorities to know my age and put me back in a foster home again. They also made sure I had some methadone to try and stop me buying heroin.

It must have been them who sent the person who ran the charity to see me. A middle-aged man who believed that everyone should be able to lead a decent life, he came to see me every day, brought me food and talked to me. I knew fairly quickly that, as we sat together talking, he was waiting for me to ask him something.

So I did.

'I don't want to be an addict,' I told him, and then taking his hand, I asked him for help.

It was he who arranged to get me into rehab.

'They will help you find work once you get clean,' he told me. 'As well as finding you somewhere to stay once you are there.'

He didn't ask my age. Instead, he just made me a cup of tea and got on the phone. He made all the arrangements with the rehab centre and drove me there. He might not realise it but he changed my life.

PART TWO

38

When we arrived at the rehab place, I could scarcely believe my eyes. I had thought that it would be like a small and bleak prison, but instead, what I saw was an enormous, beautiful house. It was old and rambling, and must once have been a private home to someone very wealthy. There were well-tended gardens, green lawns and beds of brightly coloured flowering shrubs and rose bushes. In the centre of one of the lawns was a fountain, which on closer inspection on my first exploration of the grounds, also doubled up as a fish-pond, with large coy carp lazily circling. There were benches placed throughout the gardens so that the patients could sit in solitude and enjoy the wonders of nature but also clusters of chairs where they gathered when they felt like company.

'Here we are, Amy,' said Mr Jennings, a kindly man, who was the head of the charity. 'It looks a really nice place, doesn't it?'

'It looks fantastic, more like a very expensive country hotel,' I told him.

'I expect you'll find that it does wonders for you, and who wouldn't find peace and time to reflect and recover here? I'm certain that you're going to occasionally struggle but, with the help you get here, you will recover and find a way to start afresh,' he told me, slipping a card into my hand with his contact details on it.

'Keep that and let me know later how you got on here,' he added.

After he had opened the front door for me and picked up my rucksack, the pair of us walked in together. He introduced me to the young woman on reception, said his goodbyes and, with another kind smile, he left. I had to fill in a registration form while I was in reception and then another young woman appeared and showed me around. There was a dining room, a huge lounge where a few people were sitting, a smaller one with rows of chairs, which I was told were for meetings, a well-stocked library and a games room with a pool table and a selection of board games. Then we went up the stairs, where I saw the bath and shower rooms, toilets and, last of all, after passing many other rooms, my bedroom. If I had thought it might look like a cell. I was wrong: it was a cosy place with pretty bedding, white painted furniture and even pictures on the walls.

By the end of the day, I had found that both the staff and those who were there to either stop drinking, or be clean of drugs, were friendly. After all, everyone there was either helping us to become clean or they were there because, like me, they were determined to gain sobriety and leave their addictions behind them. I was, of course, a little scared to be at this crossroads in my life but felt fortunate to have this opportunity. The rehab place only worked with those who had already taken the first step on that path themselves. While I was there, I didn't come across anyone who was there against their will. I was sure some would fall back again but, somewhere deep inside me, I knew that, with help and encouragement, I could succeed.

After I had emptied my rucksack and put everything neatly away, I was taken to see the doctor. First, I was asked more or less the same questions as the other doctors who had tried to get me off heroin, though there was one question that I hadn't been expecting.

'What is it you like about heroin, Amy? Is it because you enjoy getting high or is there another reason?'

'It takes away my sadness,' I told her.

That answer was enough for her to ask me a little more and I found myself spilling out how my mother had died before I was in my teens and my father, who I had adored, no longer wanted me in his life soon afterwards.

'Because of the heroin?'

'No, because I look exactly like my mother.'

'And that's why you liked your drugs?'

'Yes.'

More questions followed as she tried to identify the whole background to what had caused me to feel so depressed. I could see she was scribbling down notes and somehow it made me feel that she was taking me seriously and wanted to find out what made me tick.

Before I left the room, she told me that she could understand why I felt I needed drugs to help me block out the pain: 'Nearly everyone who comes in here has more than one reason why they have become addicted to the wrong things.' Then there was one other question she asked that I had never been asked during my whole time in prison, which was why I went onto methadone in the first place.

I was honest in my reply, saying that it was because I was going to Thailand, and how I had hoped it might help me win back my father's love. Then I filled her in with some more information about that trip and how everything had gone wrong there, tears filling my eyes as I explained how it had made me go back on those illegal drugs when I returned to England.

'And now?'

And now indeed. I told her exactly what I had already told Mr Jennings, the man in charge of the charity, that living on the streets had broken me, and how I wanted to be clean.

'I want to be a normal person,' I said simply.

At this she smiled before saying, 'Good for you, Amy. We're all going to work at that while you're here. Our job in this rehab house is to help you get over your depression and, by the time you leave, for you to have respect for what you've managed to achieve here. In your case, I think you will find the group therapy sessions particularly helpful.'

She then handed me a timetable and using a pink highlighter, she marked which meetings were essential. With a green highlighter, she indicated the optional ones. There were also fitness classes and yoga, which she explained also helped the body and the mind to heal and would promote good sleep and restorative relaxation.

The consultation over, she walked me back to the small meeting room, where the group therapy sessions took place. Were they helpful? They certainly were. There was such honesty in that room when others spoke about their addiction and how they had begun in the first place but it took a few sessions before I managed to talk about myself.

The one slight anger that came into the room was when I told the group how I had become addicted.

'A man older than you made you believe you were an addict after just one hit?' said one.

There was a sense of incredulity in those words and several people there said it was a terrible thing to do, especially as I was so very young. I didn't want to say any more about Pete then. Was I being protective of him? I don't think so, I just felt so stupid that I had been so trusting and gullible throughout my association with him.

I went on to tell them how I was helped by a doctor to get methadone and then went back onto heroin twice.

'That was my fault,' I told the listening room.

'Good for you,' said the person in charge of the group session. 'You mean you can't just blame other people?'

'That's right. I have to take some responsibility, don't I?'

I felt stronger after each and every one of those sessions.

39

I was quite excited when we were given jobs to do. By then I had realised that it was the patients themselves who were almost running the place. Everyone there agreed that lying around doing nothing would hardly have been good for us. To begin with, I was working in the garden. It was something I really enjoyed because it brought back some of my happy memories of helping Mum pull out weeds from her flower beds and the fresh air cleared my head a bit and made me feel more positive.

After a couple of weeks, I was asked if I would like a completely different type of job, which was dealing with the new arrivals and learning how to schedule their appointments. I was really happy to be asked to do that: for me to be chosen for such a role meant that I was trusted. Another part of the job was labelling the urine tests, which were done to make sure that no one had smuggled in drugs or alcohol. It had happened a few times, I was told, especially in cases where it was the parents or relatives who had made their relatives enter rehab reluctantly.

It was a routine test, but no one knew the exact date of it. During the time I worked there, two people were caught and the rule was clear: there were no second chances and they had to leave. That upset me a little, but I had to agree that they needed to be committed or relinquish their place to someone else on the waiting list.

While I was doing that role, one of the staff suggested, 'Maybe you could get a job in one of these rehab places when your life is back on track.'

I thought that could be an interesting prospect for me and I was told that there are quite a few people who were once patients who now work in rehab centres around the country. They could understand first-hand the issues that lead to addiction without ever looking down on those who have relapsed time and time again. I could hardly believe that, in such a short while, I had become part of what we called the HM (house management). That was when I began to feel it was the start of me becoming a law-abiding citizen and a better person: one with a future.

*　*　*

It was a couple of months later when a new volunteer arrived. He was a man well into his thirties, who everyone seemed to like. It was apparently not the first time he had come there to help and he ended up working alongside me quite often. He asked me how long I had been there and, when I replied, he asked what I was going to do when I left.

My initial answer to that was that I didn't know. I didn't tell him that I was hoping that I would be helped with finding work, as Mr Jennings from the charity had suggested, and that with a regular wage coming in I thought my next step might be to get some sort of bedsit. These thoughts I pushed to the back of my head because I knew that I was in danger of running before I could walk. When I was alone, I did try to think about what kind of job I could get, but in the meantime, I was content, as I was not only working on myself, but also learning new skills that could help me when I was ready for a life outside.

When he asked me the same question on another occasion, I decided to voice what I had been mulling over.

'I wondered if I could work in one of these rehab places – I know some patients do and I've enjoyed working here,' I told him.

In retrospect, how I wish I had never given him that answer because his reply was the beginning of me losing the confidence that I was working so hard to rebuild.

'Sounds good, Amy, but you have to have been clean for at least a year on the outside before you can apply,' was what he told me.

I still don't know whether there was any truth in that, but now I know what his plan was: to get me into his home and keep me there, which in the end he managed to do. He persuaded me to leave rehab when I had been there nearly six months, telling me there was plenty of work around where he lived and he had enough space in his flat for me to have a room there.

I agreed to go with him when his period of voluntary work came to an end. After packing my newly acquired case provided by the rehab people (using the rucksack you had on the streets was frowned upon), I left with him. I had asked my doctor and therapists if I was ready to leave and they agreed I was.

In all the times ahead with that man, I was subjected to many sorts of degradation but my deceitful friend remained my sworn enemy and I have never taken drugs again.

That was the day I walked out of my safe haven, not just into loneliness but into hell.

40

I realise now that, when James started to take an interest in me, he already knew I had no family that I could escape to. He had also worked out that, if I stayed in the rehab for a while longer, I would have got my whole future completely mapped out. The people in charge would have contacted my sponsor, Mr Jennings, who would never have let me go back to the streets and would have helped me get myself set up with a good job and somewhere to live. James must have seen that the jobs I was doing in the centre were giving me confidence and a foundation to assist me in becoming an independent and productive member of society.

James had also done his research about Mr Jennings and already knew that he was a well-off man, who was dedicated to helping vulnerable adolescents. He himself was the opposite sort of man to Mr Jennings – he wanted to prevent my life from improving further and to take me away from the healthy environment of the rehab altogether and make me his puppet. Without a family of my own, he had finally found the right girl; one who he could control. The one who after a short while would do whatever he wanted her to. All he had to do was persuade her to leave this place, which is exactly what he did. He knew I had nowhere to go to once I left, so what did he do? He offered me a room in his large flat.

'What about rent?' I asked tentatively.

'When you get a job, you can chip in, Amy,' he said with a warm smile. He also told me not to tell anyone that I would be staying in his flat – 'They might think that I can always be relied upon to put people up, but I'm selective, there's not everyone I would want to stay.'

That made me feel a little special.

'I like to help people like you, Amy, ones who have ambition,' he added.

Help them get to a point where they want to kill themselves might have been a better description, I can confidently say now.

Sadly, that was not a thought that entered my head then.

So, I told the staff I was leaving. I had heard about a good job I could get and a friend was going to put me up. They congratulated me, though I was also asked if I was certain that I was ready to leave rehab.

'I'm ready, I know I am,' I told them glibly.

41

James's large flat had pale cream walls, which were half-covered in huge pieces of modern art in vibrant, primary colours. I was told they were painted by a well-known artist who fetched high prices and exhibited widely in the UK and internationally. They must have cost a pretty penny and, although I responded to their enormity, I had to ask myself whether I liked them. In truth, I thought they were a bit disturbing. On either side of the fireplace, which had an imitation log fire in it, were two four-seater black leather settees. Now those I really didn't like the look of – not one cushion or throw in sight, they were hardly inviting. It might have looked like a rich man's home but, to me, there was something cold and clinical about the place.

The kitchen, where everything in it appeared to be made of stainless steel, was the tidiest one I had ever seen. Every item was stored in cupboards, even down to the kettle and the toaster, which told me it would be unwise for me ever to leave anything out on one of those pristine surfaces, like a used cup or plate, let alone a smear of butter or a toast crumb. I suspected it would also be frowned upon if a book was temporarily laid aside on a table or on the seat of one of the sofas.

For the first couple of weeks everything seemed all right. James was rather abrupt when he spoke to me, but I could go walking round the neighbourhood and I could read a book taken from the small shelf of books, which somewhat strangely, were arranged by colour and size. But I missed working and more than once I asked him if there were any jobs he knew of, so that I could apply.

'Not yet,' was the brief answer.

Somehow, I didn't dare ask how long it would be until I could get an interview. After I had been there for nearly two weeks, I began to wish I had stayed in rehab, although, as James repeatedly told me, I couldn't have stayed there forever, which made me push those thoughts aside.

I offered to do some cooking for him. I knew I wasn't that good – my opportunities to learn had been limited – but I could still manage some of the simpler things I had learnt in the rehab kitchens. The answer to that was a firm, 'No, thank you,' as he showed me all the ready meals in his freezer. All I had to do was warm them up and serve them, put the dishes in the dishwasher and make sure there was not one smear left on the glass dining table after we had eaten.

A few days after this conversation, he told me about a big family party that he wanted to take me to. On hearing this, I felt my cheeks flush a little. Going to a party didn't really sound much fun to me, not when I wouldn't know anyone there. It had been so long since I had been out with groups of people, this invitation made me feel a little uneasy. Especially as I hardly had anything suitable to wear – as you can imagine, there was not much call for party clothes when I was on the streets.

I'm sure then he knew that I wasn't confident about going. I thought that he was being kind when he told me he was taking me shopping for the event. 'I'm going to take you to a shop I know, where I can get you a nice new outfit,' he said. 'You can't wear those old things of yours where we're going.'

I wanted to say that I wouldn't mind staying behind, but there was something in his manner that told me to try and sound grateful.

What did I say about control earlier? I said that there is more than one way of stripping away the layers of a person's confidence. With James, this was his first major step: to choose what he wanted me to wear, not what I would like to be dressed in. That shopping spree was very different to the fun outings I had done with Mum, her friend Anne or any of the friends my own age. With them, there was always lots of laughter and compliments before we treated ourselves to coffee and cake afterwards. Shopping with James didn't bear any resemblance to those days.

He was the one with the money, so it was his right to choose what he liked enough for me to be seen out with him wearing. Or at least that was how I saw it at the time. When we walked into the shop, which was the smartest one I had ever been into, he told me to take a seat and wait while he explained to the shop owner, not the assistant who initially approached us, what he was looking for. I could tell by her expression that it was not the first time he had been there. She must have had a good idea of what it was he wanted because, within minutes, she had selected three dresses for him to look at. Each one was low-cut with thin straps that went over the shoulders. He fingered the fabric of all three of them.

'That one,' he said decisively, selecting a silvery garment with a floaty skirt, but I could see there was not much fabric above the waist. Hardly the ideal choice for a girl who liked to wear jeans and T-shirts. Having injected in my arms for so long, I always wore long sleeves and I was acutely aware that the veins in my arms still looked damaged. While on the street, I had found those veins were collapsing and, like many users, I had switched to injecting my groin, where the veins are bigger – a horrifying bit of knowledge I learned on the street. In the fitting room, I was careful to keep my arms out of sight of the shop owner as I got changed into the dress to make sure it fitted.

'Good thing you're young with a nice figure, because you can't wear a bra with this one,' she told me, zipping it up.

If there wasn't much material at the front, there was hardly any at the back of the dress either. Just the thought of walking out of the changing room in something so skimpy made me blush. Luckily, I didn't need to: the dress fitted me perfectly, but it was just not my style. I could hardly tell James that I didn't feel comfortable wearing it as he was already waving his credit card in front of the owner.

The next stop was a shoe shop, and again, it was James who said what it was he wanted. By now, I was lost for words and looked on helplessly. I had to try on the pair of shoes he had chosen. With their high, thin heels, I doubted if I would ever manage to walk in them. As I took a few tentative steps around the shop, I wobbled badly.

'You can practise walking in them when you're back in the flat,' he told me after observing my discomfort.

Back home, he sat and watched as I began practising in my shoes, insisting I wore the dress too – 'They make you look taller and that means you look a bit thinner. That full skirt hides the plumpness around your stomach as well.'

So much for that boutique owner telling me I had a good figure! I knew I was short, but I hadn't thought I was over-weight until then. *I'd better do some exercises*, I told myself, *and cut out the toast and marmalade too.*

The next thing he wanted to sort out was make-up, which I hardly ever wore much of. I had always preferred the natural look and recently there had been no money for that sort of thing. He took me to the cosmetics counter of a department store and had them do my make-up after telling them that I would be attending an evening event. I barely owned a lip balm, so when the make-up artist finally achieved the look he wanted, he purchased everything she had used to turn me into the painted doll that stared back at me in the mirror.

Afterwards, he told me, 'You'd better spend some time practising making your face look as good as this before we go. See how it makes your eyes look a little larger and your lips a bit thicker? As for that hair of yours, no pony-tail or having it straggling down your shoulders, I want it up in a chignon.'

I almost told him then that my thick hair was always

admired but somehow I managed to keep quiet, yet again unable to find the words.

'So, make sure you start practising that as well, Amy. After all, you haven't got anything else to do, have you?'

I hadn't, but how I wished I had.

That was the beginning of him making me feel inferior.

* * *

It was a few days later when, feeling half-naked in the dress that showed the outline of my nipples through the thin fabric, he drove us to the big house where the party was being held. Before we left, he had examined me closely, making me turn round so that he could study my appearance from all angles. Then he nodded and told me I looked all right. Not that I felt it – after all, 'all right' was hardly the most encouraging compliment.

On the drive there he hardly spoke to me and, when we reached the house, all he had to do was flick a button on his key ring for the gates to slide open. I noticed there were a couple of men near the doors. Recognising James straight away, they smiled in our direction and stepped forward to open the car doors to let us out before one of them drove the vehicle to a parking area. What I realised some time later was that they were bodyguards and their job was to make sure that no uninvited strangers could follow a car in.

As I walked in nervously with James, I glanced around and noted with a sinking heart that I was by far the youngest person there. I also felt acutely self-conscious in my dress. The worst part of the first few minutes was that James suddenly announced that he had to talk to his family. I expected him to take me with him and introduce me but he didn't. Instead, he instructed me to wander round and introduce myself to people. As you can imagine, the thought of this was terrifying to me and so I blinked at him in horror.

'Not difficult, is it, Amy, seeing as you are all dressed up? Everyone here is as well and they will be friendly, I promise you,' he told me coldly.

He might have thought that, but now I suspect that he was certain that I wouldn't have enough confidence to walk up to groups of complete strangers who were chatting away to people they obviously knew; strangers who mostly appeared to be twice my age. Hardly any of the guests caught my eye and none of them invited me over to join their group. There were a few girls who I suspected were not that much older than me, standing next to men who looked just about old enough to be their grandfathers. Like me, they, too, were wearing low-cut dresses and wore similar stilettos on their feet. Their jewellery looked expensive as well. Judging from the cars outside – a Mercedes, a couple of Rolls and several very sleek sports cars – I guessed that the men at this party were more than just a little well off.

It didn't take that long for me to conclude that, wealthy or not, these men hadn't been born that way. Beneath their tailored garments were men I came to know who were, if not crooks, not entirely honest. By then, I could scarcely believe that for the second time in my life, I had found myself in a group of people that I was eager to get away from.

There were waitresses dressed in black and white who brought round trays of canapés. And others who carried round glasses of wine or champagne. I wished I was one of them instead of being an awkward girl on her own, wearing such a low-cut dress – I felt like an imposter.

I hadn't expected to enjoy the party, but it was even worse than I had imagined in my wildest dreams. There was something about the women near me, who made me feel that I wouldn't be made to feel welcome if I dared to go over and tried to talk to them. They had seen me come in with James and must have noticed that he was nowhere to be seen. I caught them looking over at me and taking me in before whispering to each other and then sniggering.

Eventually, one of them walked over to me with a smug little grin on her face. 'Don't tell me you're James's latest little girlfriend,' she said loudly enough for all her friends to hear, causing even more sniggers.

When I replied that he was just a friend, I received a dismissive shrug.

'Not for long, love,' she said before she turned and walked away.

As for the men there, I cringed when I saw their hungry eyes looking me up and down. One of them came over and made some small talk with me. He told me that he was a friend of James and the family and I felt grateful that at last someone was talking to me, but he must have got tired of my limited conversation because he soon returned to his inner circle. Walking around the party on my own was hardly something anyone would have enjoyed, no matter how confident they might have been. I had already been feeling extremely nervous and now, with these setbacks, I just wanted to go and wait in the car.

I can remember us finally leaving after what seemed like hours and me feeling such relief that I was at last out of there.

* * *

I didn't have a clue what was in store for me or what game James was going to play once we got back to his flat. The first round of insults began almost as the front door clicked shut and he turned on me.

'I saw you stuffing your face all night,' he said angrily. 'And I heard that you were knocking back champagne as though you were used to it. Which anyone there would know, you weren't. And did you actually try and talk to my family? No, Amy, you did not!'

'I didn't know which people were your family,' I just about managed to splutter out, for he had never introduced them to me or pointed them out. Nor did I think for one moment that he had been watching me.

'I didn't see you trying to talk to anyone. You just looked like a sullen child. And to think how much money I've spent on you,' he continued.

I tried to tell him it wasn't true; I had spoken to people (well, two of them at least). I had only had three small glasses of bubbles over the whole evening and I hadn't eaten a lot either. Apart from anything else, I was too nervous to eat and I was afraid that, if I had more than three glasses of champagne, I might easily become drunk and embarrass him.

'Now, look in the mirror on that wall and tell me what you see,' he said coldly.

'Me in a silvery dress,' I naively told him.

'What *I* see, Amy, is a big fat, ugly, stupid bitch. Now stay looking… Say it, say your name and then I want to hear those words I have just said to you.'

I could hardly believe what I was hearing and so I just stood stock-still, staring at my reflection in the mirror, now wearing a shocked expression.

'Say it, Amy!' he snapped. 'I'll give you thirty seconds.'

I glared at him then.

'What?! Amy, do you want to be back on the streets, selling your little body for drugs?' he sneered.

Stunned, I gasped at that insult. I had never even thought of doing that, not once, I told him.

Oh, how he laughed at me then.

'Say it or I might just throw you back out.'

That was the first time I gave in to his commands and, to my shame, I now found myself standing in front of the mirror, verbally insulting myself. It was almost like a mantra of self-harm and it didn't take long before I was forced to do it again and again. The next time I had to stand there for over thirty minutes and the following one for over an hour. I did my best not to cry each time, for there were other things happening to me that were far worse.

It was about two days later when I found out the real reason that he had brought me there: he wanted a child and I was the person he had chosen to make pregnant and provide him with one.

Wanting to appear as firm as I could, I stood up, drew my shoulders back and said, 'No, absolutely not! I'm too young to have a baby. Anyhow, I want to get a job and earn enough to pay rent and look after myself.'

'I heard you, but I've already told you what *I* want from you so don't repeat all that, Amy,' James said in reply.

But I did.

That was when a clenched fist landed as hard as it could in my stomach, leaving me doubled up and gasping for breath. At that point came the realisation that this was the start of his second method of control. Shockwaves overwhelmed me, for no one, not even those policemen who had hurt my wrist so badly when I was arrested on the street, had ever attacked me like that. I was shaking with fright. What sort of person had I moved in with? I seriously thought that he might kill me. In fact, I was lucky he didn't. There were times later on when he was not far off from doing just that. And times when

I thought I would rather be dead than have to deal with his behaviour.

Through my shock, I heard his calm, cold voice telling me to go into the bedroom.

'Get undressed in there, you hear me, Amy?'

So I did. I just about managed to crawl into the room.

He came in behind me, and because I wasn't undressing fast enough for him, he pulled the rest of my clothes off, picked me up and threw me on the bed. I could feel his hot breath on my face, his hands squeezing my breasts so hard I was in agony, but not as much as when he forced himself into me and then banged away for what seemed like hours. No sooner had he come than he stopped for a few minutes before starting over – again and then again. He left me in the early hours and then I lay curled up and clutching my bruised and aching stomach, tears streaming down my face.

I became his prisoner. I had to give him the date my period was due. Up until then, he dragged me into the bedroom every night. When my period eventually came, telling us both that I wasn't pregnant, he slapped me across the face.

'Useless little whore, aren't you?' he spat and then he hit me again.

At least he didn't want to come near me over those few days.

No sooner had my period come to an end than he was back in my bed.

* * *

Four miserable weeks later, when even taking a few steps around the flat proved painful, I had to tell him that my period hadn't come. At this, I saw the gloating look of pleasure on his face: 'It had better be because you're with child now.' Despite this threat, I almost hoped so too – at least then he wouldn't want to come into my bed or hit me so often because I might miscarry if he did.

Eager to keep control, James had already bought a pregnancy testing kit from the chemist. Catching hold of my arm, he frogmarched me to the bathroom and made me pee in front of him. Silently, we watched until we saw the blue line appear.

'Well, Amy, now you have my baby inside you,' he announced.

I wanted to say 'mine too', but common sense told me not to.

The one good thing about being pregnant was that James did as I had thought he might: he ceased having sex with me or using his fists. This was only to prevent a miscarriage, though. My morning sickness was something else he hated. He was always telling me that he could hear me throwing up and accused me of sticking my fingers down my throat just to annoy him. He also ordered me to put make-up on – he didn't want to look at my pasty face.

Now that he knew I was pregnant, he gave me what he considered to be the right foods for a woman in my condition – 'Lots of vitamins in that,' he would say as he pushed a plate of tasteless mush in front of me. It must have been frustrating for him not to be able to punch me in the stomach, but he had sorted out other ways of punishing me. If I had done something he didn't like, such as burping or, even worse, farting, which pregnancy often causes, his face would go red with rage. It would be then that he would make me eat on the floor, like an animal.

A bowl would go down under the table.

'Eat it,' he urged as he pushed me down to my knees.

He would force me to stay there, pushing food into my mouth with my fingers while his feet rested on my behind. Those were some of the times he seemed to enjoy most – he was always keen to find new ways of humiliating me and never seemed to tire of his silly, cruel games.

At least during the time that my pregnancy was showing, quite often he went out alone. The relief as the door closed behind him was immense. I would try and rest, but the fear of what he might do when he came back never left me.

Why didn't I run then?

Simple: there was nowhere to run to. The people he knew would find me in five minutes, he threatened.

And still I believed him.

43

On the evenings when James decided to stay in, he found a different way of hurting me and that was enough to muddle up all my memories. I don't know how he had gathered so much information about me. I can only assume that his voluntary work gave him access to my confidential file. He had also been sitting in on some of the therapy sessions when I had told the group about how I felt about losing my mum. That gave him ammunition to work with so he could play games with my mind. He must have filed away those revelations so that he could use them as weapons against me. When it suited him he could repeat every word of what he had heard within the group verbatim.

Often, he would start this one-way conversation with me after we had eaten. With my pregnancy advancing, he could tell that I wanted to go to bed and rest, but that was not something he would allow when he was in. Not when he wanted to mentally batter me.

He frequently began by running my mother down –

'Heard everything about her being a retard. Just like you, wasn't she?'

'No,' I said, flustered.

He then threw the next insult at me: 'Well, she would have been one with that clot in that small brain of hers.'

My whole body would stiffen then, partly with anguish that he could spit out such horrid words and partly for fear of what he might say or do next. I couldn't help it, it made me cringe and I still expected him to jump up and swing his fist at me, even though he was now using words to hurt me.

'Oh, you're so pathetic, crying about dead people, aren't you?' he brayed before taking another verbal swipe at me. 'I heard you in rehab, bawling about your mum's death. Everyone was so bored by you. "I don't have any family," I kept hearing you say. And I'll tell you something else, if your mum hadn't died, she'd be sitting in her own shit by now, unable to say a word that would make any sense. Now, Amy, why don't you keep that picture in your head?'

I know now that his intention was to make me forget all the benefits of the therapy and become the damaged person I had been all over again.

But it wasn't over yet...

'I can understand why your father wants nothing to do with you. Can't say I blame him for fleeing to Thailand. He must be really sorry he didn't make your mum abort you. He hates the sight of you now, doesn't he, Amy?'

I had nothing to say then, so I remained silent, fighting back the tears.

'Now cheer up, Amy, I've done you a big favour. I decided

you needed help to forget your past. So, what did I do? I went through all your belongings and found these...'

From behind his back, he produced the couple of photos of Mum and me that I always kept with me. Right in front of me, he ripped them to shreds. 'That's them gone,' he announced with that loathsome smirk of his. 'Now here's another thing I found that you're never going to need again...' To my horror, I saw that he was holding up the card with Mr Jennings' contact details on it. The one person who I could have asked for help. At least that's what I had planned to do when I gave birth to my baby in the hospital.

As for the landline in the house, he made sure it was locked whenever he went out. There would be no trying to find phone numbers.

That's when complete and utter despair hit me.

44

The months went slowly by and my body changed shape. When I was pretty large, I could feel my baby's movements. James might have seen the baby as his alone, but I saw my bulge and I knew the little person in there that would be mine. How I wished I could just walk out of the hospital where James had booked me a private room to somewhere safe; somewhere my baby and I could be free of him.

Having a private room was not a thoughtful treat, which is what he called it. It was to stop me meeting anyone else there. For me it was another part of the prison he had locked me in.

Over those next months, James made me believe that he knew all the hospital staff and the doctor I would be seeing was a friend of his. Was all that true? Looking back, I doubt it. The doctor knew him because, apparently, I was not the only young woman he had made pregnant. Which didn't mean that they were remotely friends. Unfortunately, I was by then so under his control that I daren't try to find out if the staff really knew him. Otherwise I could have asked for help, but I was far too scared to do so.

I can remember giving birth. No need to describe all the pushing I had to do. Every other mother knows what that's like, and how the moment a tiny baby is put into our arms, all the memories of pain disappear to be replaced by surges of love. To me, it made no difference as to who the father was: she was mine.

'My daughter,' was all James kept saying when I brought her home. I had to feed her away from him and change her nappies in my room as well – that was the part of having her he didn't want to see.

It seemed one child was not enough for him, though: he wanted another. And he refused to wait for my body to recover before he was in my bed again. This time, I pleaded with him not to force himself on me but that only seemed to make him more violent. He must have been scared when I haemorrhaged after one particularly vicious assault, though, with the prospect of a dead body in his home. That time, he called for an ambulance – I had lost so much blood that I was kept in hospital for three days.

He paid for someone to stay in his flat and look after my baby until I came home. I was devastated not to be with her, but not in any fit state to argue.

I've no idea what excuses he gave to the hospital staff.

Having spotted the bruises on my legs, the doctor gently asked me if I had been attacked. If only I hadn't been so scared of James, I could have told him the truth – but I didn't. I just made up some silly excuse about being clumsy. My fear then was that he would keep my baby and throw me out. She had been switched to formula in my absence, so he didn't need me to look after her.

So how long did I stay with James after that episode? Four years – I still can't believe I stayed that long. During that time, my baby was christened at the local church. How I wanted to go – I was waiting for the opportunity to just take her and run. She went from baby to toddler, and then small child; she heard the beatings, my cries and his angry shouts. I knew it was having a damaging effect on her and I felt terrible. Her nightmares started before she turned four.

It was when she reached four and a half that I escaped.

I'm convinced that he never thought I would leave. She had started going to a nursery school and one lucky morning came when he couldn't take her. He ordered a taxi and told me it was my turn. That was the morning I took a couple of twenty-pound notes I had stashed under my bedroom carpet. It was the last of the money from that stolen wallet, which I had kept hidden from him.

When I climbed into the taxi with my daughter, I was shaking with fear. I told the driver that there had been a change of plan and he was to take me to a station in another town. Then I waited anxiously. Would he refuse? After all, it was James who had the account with the taxi firm.

All he said was, 'That's OK.'

An hour later, I was on a train. I might have felt sick with nerves that James would make sure to find me, but I also knew where I could get help. I took out my phone and made the call using the new SIM card I had bought in the newspaper shop at the station.

Then I knew where I was going.

45

When I finally stepped off the train, a young and good-looking man put his hand out to help me. 'Hello, Amy,' he said before bending down a little so that he could look into my daughter's face as he greeted her as well. Although usually shy, she looked straight at him and smiled.

Now where did he come from?

The answer is that he had been in and out of my life since I was around eight.

It was the summer of 2004 and the beginning of school holidays when I met him for the first time. Both the warmth of the sun and being free of school made us want to play outside. There were quite a few children around my age group near where I lived. If we were not in the same classes at school, all our birthday parties meant that we had got know each other pretty well.

There was one boy a couple of years older than me who I didn't see as a friend. In fact, I never wanted to be anywhere near him. He had a knack of chasing after me, calling me names and, if he caught me, his little podgy fingers busy themselves pinching my arms. Well, little boys can be mean, can't they? I've since heard that he's now a happily married man with a couple of children of his own, who adore him. Back then, though, he was a nasty piece of work.

The day I met Ryan was when that young bully grabbed my arm and began his pinching. I tried to slap him with my free hand and he tried to push me away, which caused me to land on my backside. So there I sat inelegantly on the ground weeping while the other boys laughed at me. It was then out of the corner of my eye that I saw the figure of another boy rushing over.

Gentle hands pulled me up. As he dabbed at my eyes with his fingertips, he told me not to cry any more.

'I want to go home,' I said, still snivelling.

'I'll take you,' he said and, together, we walked over to my house.

'Sounds like a nice boy,' said Mum when I came in and told her what had happened.

'I like him,' I said.

At this, she smiled and gave me a warm hug, then some fruit juice, which made me forget all about being pushed over. But I didn't forget the boy who had helped me.

During those summer holidays, there were days when Mum took me out and weekends when Dad would drive us all to the coast. There was also a holiday where the three of us travelled to another country on a plane. In between all of that, I would still join the other children in playing all sorts of games outside. I would always be on the lookout for Ryan, and the moment I saw him, I would leave my friends and run over to him. He never seemed to mind me following him about during that summer; he would smile at me and we would chat away.

All too soon, the school holidays ended and then we were back in school. Gradually, I saw less and less of him as he was in a different class to me. Then about a year later, he left our school to go to the senior one and I hardly ever saw him then. I think by then my little crush had faded, though.

* * *

The next time I spoke to Ryan was when I was in senior school. One day I needed the toilet and so off I went, only to find that the door leading to the loos was locked. I was so annoyed that I began kicking the door and swearing at it. It was then that I heard a voice behind say, 'I've got a key.' I spun round and laughed when I saw it was Ryan, who by then had grown quite tall and good-looking. He got up from the little alcove near the door where he had been sitting.

'It's the girls' loo,' I said. 'How come you've got the key?'

'I pinched it and the boys' one too off the teacher's desk,' he told me.

I doubt if that was true. It was more likely that , as a prefect at the school, he had been asked to go and unlock the toilets in case someone had locked them by mistake.

I recognised him straight away but I could tell that he didn't know then that I was the girl he once helped. Or if he did know, he hid it quite well. He leant against the door and asked me my name but I just shook my head. I saw myself as a teenager so I hardly wanted him to remember that tearful child sat on her behind or how I had once followed him around like a puppy who has lost its collar.

'I need to get in,' I told him.

He unlocked the door and opened it for me, then tried to follow me in.

'What do you think you're doing, coming into a girls' loo?' I asked, though I couldn't help grinning.

'I think you're beautiful,' he said. 'You can't blame me for trying to get to know you, now can you?'

'Then wait till we're in the playground,' I told him.

Another grin and he walked away.

Ryan did as I told him to, which was to come up to me in the playground. We began to be friends then, though there was always an undercurrent of something more serious. I liked him a lot – he was fun and I knew that I could trust him too.

In our early teens, however, there was a reason for his feelings about me to change. It was when he saw me with Pete that he began to ask questions that I found hard to answer. He had heard the rumours about Pete dealing drugs – something he disapproved of – and I can't say I blame him for wanting to know if I was doing drugs too. I denied it but eventually he found out that I was injecting myself with heroin – he had seen the marks on my arms that I tried my best to hide. By then, I was injecting my groin as it was easier to find a vein there, but still those marks remained. Ryan didn't want to mix with anyone who took drugs and he wanted to know if that was the reason why I was meeting up with Pete.

'Don't tell me you're a junkie,' he said sadly.

He made it clear then that we were not going to be any more than casual friends unless I stopped seeing Pete and got myself clean. By that time I thought it was too late – I was back on drugs shortly after I returned from Thailand.

So how come he was at the station?

I had managed to contact him.

The one place I could go to on my own was the library. Thank goodness for James's OCD – he didn't want piles of children's books lying around any more than he wanted toys in any of the rooms. That was the reason I was able to persuade him to let me take Trinity to the library. I was only allowed to bring back two books: one for me and another that I could read to her. James would drop me off there so I could take our daughter in and help her choose a book with plenty of pictures in it. Then I'd grab something else for me to read as quickly as possible.

What hadn't occurred to James was that there were computers in the library that I could use. There were a couple of people I tried to find online but couldn't, but I knew Ryan had gone to the library to look up Pete, and yes, my heart jumped when I saw his photo.

Would he help me?

Remember that little boy who helped you up when you were eight. The boy who stopped you being bullied, I told myself firmly.

I nervously messaged him on Facebook, telling him that I needed help but would understand if he didn't reply and that I wouldn't have access to a computer again for a week.

It was nearly a week later when I was able to go to the

library again. As I checked for any messages, I found Ryan's reply: he had written straight back to say that he had never forgotten me and that yes, he would help.

It took a few more visits to the library – I couldn't spend too much time in there – to tell him a lot about me needing to get away from James.

He actually offered to come and get us, It almost felt unreal, to have someone care and want to help, but I told him that would be too risky – I would just have to wait until I could get away. I already sensed that something was going to happen to allow my escape – and it did.

As we walked from the station, he took hold of my hand.

'You'll be safe with me,' he told me. 'You will *both* be safe.'

As we walked, I felt the clouds of despair lift from my shoulders and float away.

Acknowledgements from Amy Jones

I want to dedicate this book to the man who named me Fallen Angel, the man I've loved all those years, who saved me not only from a living hell but from myself: Ryan Jones, I'm talking to you. And to our three beautiful girls: each day that passes, I see more of me in all of you, which, to be honest, terrifies me. Don't make the choices I made, don't give in and always say no – I made those mistakes so you can learn from me. My eldest knows what I was and most things about my life, but the day will come when I have to tell the others. I love my girls – thank you for saving me.

People think that, once you stop taking the drugs and your rattle is done, you're cured, which is why most families break down and the addict drifts away. I may be clean now but I was – and always will be – a heroin addict. Phoenix House saved my life and gave me my first proper home in years.

Dad, you died the week before I married. Somewhere you

should have been was by my side, walking me down the aisle and giving me away, bursting with pride. You gave up on me when I needed you most but I still had the most amazing childhood anyone could have and you gave me the world. I was your princess: a daddy's girl. Nobody meant more to you than me, but in the end, you saw my mum looking at you through me each day. I didn't cry – why would I when you died long ago? But you were once my hero, and that little girl cried. My mum, Mary Pearson, was the best mum anyone could wish for: thank you for being my mum, I'm sorry I let you down but I hope I've now made you proud. I love people saying I look like you – I never saw it at the time but I'm your double as a teen. Thanks for all the parties, the Christmases, the holidays… Most of all, thank you for being my mum: I love you x

Ryan A381R, you really are my happy ever after.

Callum, my brother-in-law who serves in the army as a Grenadier Guard, we are so proud of you. Les and Kathleen Jones, you raised a man to be proud of – thank you.

And finally, Toni Maguire, who not only believed in me and helped me through difficult times, but treated me like a person and never judged. To me that means a hell of a lot.

Any addict that's reading this, I'm talking to you: you can beat it, you can win the battle. I know there's nothing worse than withdrawing and it's so hard not to just give in to feel better. If that's the case, get a methadone script, then every day you will feel normal with no withdrawal symptoms. I know that a few people reading my story will relate to it and see themselves in me, in how I lived, and will go and get clean because of this book. Or at least I hope they will – if it's just one person, then all I've been through will have been worth it. Parents, keep a watch on your daughters' boyfriends – you need to stop it carrying on. At twelve, I was given heroin by a lad I'd met who was older than me and played the biggest part of all in destroying my life. You know who you are, and yes, you're to blame. Yes, I blame it all on you: you gave me heroin, knowing what would happen, and no, I won't forgive you. I'll never regret the way I destroyed you, but always know that, though you took my life, I took your heart.

From Toni

Amy – From the very first message you sent me, I admired your courage. I knew, over the next few months as you shared with me details of your past, that none of it could have been easy. In your story I saw a brave child who turned out to be a remarkable adult.

I would like to thank three people who have helped me on my journey: my editor, Ciara Lloyd, my copyeditor, Jane Donovan, and Barbara Levy, who has been my loyal agent for nearly twenty years. Thanks to you all.

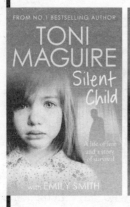 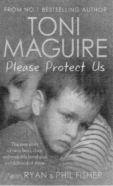 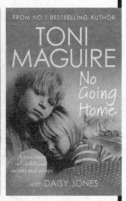